I1039147

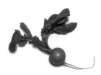

"*After reading* **The Living Foods Lifestyle**, *I know Ann Wigmore lives on. Brenda Cobb not only captures the spirit, but creates a highly organized system for integrating a holistic, simple approach that fits into modern lifestyles leading to energy, perfect weight, beauty and longer life. This cutting-edge book is a must for every home.*"

- Viktoras Kulvinskas, M.S., bestselling author, **Survival Into The 21st Century**; and co-founder, with Dr. Ann Wigmore of the world-famous Hippocrates Health Institute

"*Brenda Cobb's story is truly an inspiration. It's a true testament of how one individual's inner transformation can radiate out and positively shift the lives of thousands of people. Brenda is an outstanding leader in the Living Foods grass-roots revolution. In her amazing book, you will find hope and wonder as recipes, testimonials and common sense are successfully integrated into a simple, elegant healing program.*"

– David Wolfe, author, **The Sunfood Diet Success System** and **Eating For Beauty**

"*Please place this book on the altar of your health library. It's an excellent description of how the natural laws of living can help you regain your health. It says in words what Brenda Cobb has shown in her own life's healing and also at her wonderful, 'hands-on' Living Foods Institute in Atlanta, Georgia. I congratulate her and I'm sure so would Ann (Wigmore).*"

– Dean Martens, M.H., President & Founder, Herbs of Light, Inc.

"*Through the Living Foods Institute and her life's example, Brenda Cobb is an inspiring role model of how to achieve a healthy, Living and raw foods lifestyle here in the Atlanta metropolitan area. Those of us whose lives she has touched owe her a great debt of gratitude.*"

– Coretta Scott King

"*Brenda's gift was to become ill, then responsible, then well, and now, most importantly, to share it with the world. Within the pages of this book you will learn how easy it is to gain a full, productive and happy life. Congratulations Brenda!*"

– Brian Clement, Director Hippocrates Health Institute

HEALTH · BEAUTY · ENERGY · JOY · ABUNDANCE · PEACE

The

LIVING
FOODS
LIFESTYLE

*An inspiring guide filled with remarkable stories
and delicious raw and Living Foods recipes.*

BRENDA COBB

THE LIVING FOODS LIFESTYLE
By Brenda Cobb

This book is sold for information purposes only. The author, editor and/or publisher are not accountable or responsible for the use or misuse of the information contained in this book. This book is not intended as medical advice and the author, editor and publisher are making no claims that this Lifestyle or way of eating will alleviate health problems. We do not recommend that anyone follow this Lifestyle as a treatment for any symptom or disease however minor or serious. The therapeutic procedures in this book are based on the training, personal experiences and research of the author. The testimonials in this book were given freely and without coercion or compensation. Because each person and situation are unique, the author, editor and publisher urge the reader to check with a qualified health professional before using any procedure, if there is any question as to its appropriateness or if you have particular health concerns. Because there is always some risk involved, the author, editor, publisher and/or distributors of this book are not responsible for any adverse detoxification effects or consequences resulting from the use of any suggestions, preparations or procedures described hereafter. The author, editor and publisher are not responsible for detoxification or side effects that may occur from the use or suggestion of any of the material contained herein. When a person who has been eating cooked food switches to a Living Foods diet, it is highly likely they will experience detoxification side effects. This is a normal part of the process and necessary when removing toxins from the body. Please do not use this book if you are unwilling to assume the risk.

Cover design and book layout: Alston Anderson, Anderson/Griffin
Cover photo, chapter head photos and author's photo: Jane L. Holmes
Editor: Shannon Wilder

ISBN 10: 0-9721490-0-7
ISBN 13: 978-0-9721490-0-6

Fourth Edition: April 2009

Printed in the United States of America by Falcon Books.

Published by:
Living Soul Publishing
1530 Dekalb Ave. NE, Ste. E
Atlanta, Georgia 30307
www.livingfoodsinstitute.com
(404) 524-4488

DEDICATION

This book is dedicated to the memory of my father, Harry Burnette.
Daddy, your love and support give me strength every day. You are my special
guardian angel, and I feel you all around me. Thank you for teaching me how to
be strong and telling me how I could be anything, accomplish anything or
do anything I set my mind to. I believed every word and
I am living those words today. I miss you
and I love you very much.

A NOTE FROM THE AUTHOR

IN HONOR OF ANN WIGMORE

The information about the Living Foods Lifestyle is not my original idea. It was first developed and taught by the great healer, Ann Wigmore. Only the personal story and results I have achieved from following the Living Foods Lifestyle are original to this work. All information about the Living Foods Lifestyle contained in this book was gathered from other works by Ann Wigmore and all credits for the development of this work go exclusively to her and her colleagues. It is with great respect and a deep sense of honor that I pass along her teachings – and my personal experiences – to the reader.

Brenda Cobb
Atlanta, Georgia
May 2002

TABLE
OF CONTENTS

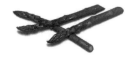

FOREWORD

As a fellow 100 percent raw/Living Foodist and medical doctor board-certified in preventive medicine, I applaud and praise Brenda Cobb for this outstanding work, *The Living Foods Lifestyle.*

This book is a must read for all who are interested in:
- "true" preventive medicine
- preventing and reversing disease
- outstanding longevity and life extension
- emotional poise and sexual potency
- vitality and mental clarity
- great digestion and assimilation
- optimizing your health

Brenda has presented this effort in a clear, effective, organized, sincere, powerful and intense way that includes:
- great inspiration and motivation to empower you
- fantastic real life testimonial that provides a beacon of hope for overcoming any health challenge
- practical experience and instructions explained in detail so you can apply these principles to your life now
- important, clear presentation of raw and Living Foods theory.

In this modern age, as we are experiencing epidemics of cancer and heart and artery disease, as well as a long list of other chronic degenerative diseases (diabetes, arthritis, auto-immune, Alzheimer's, chronic fatigue and more) we must take advantage of the Living Foods Lifestyle as presented in these pages.

From a historical perspective, we all must realize that humans (and animals) have evolved magnificently over millions of years as raw and Living Foods consumers without stoves, microwave ovens or crock pots. Our ancestors didn't have canned soup, boxed macaroni and cheese, hamburgers and French fries, or pasteurized milk on the menu. And judging from archaeological fossil records, our prehistoric human counterparts did not suffer from the physical deterioration that we (as well as domesticated animals) are now experiencing on our current diet of processed, refined, adulterated and cooked food.

Also, consider that every living organism on planet earth eats 100 percent raw or Living Foods – not 99 percent, not 70 percent, not 50 percent ... but 100 percent! There's only one organism that tampers with its food – man. We're the only animal on the planet that has decided to cook its food.

You might ask why does the body function so much better on a fresh food diet? And what does cooking (and processing) actually do to the nutritional value of the food?

- Heating food beyond 105 degrees Fahrenheit destroys the enzymes that all foods contain. These enzymes help us pre-digest our foods, and manufacturing them internally robs the body of energy and reduces our capacity to manufacture enzymes for other vital functions such as maintaining our immune systems.

- Heating food destroys many vitamins that were originally present. Vitamins in pill form are a poor substitute for the real thing.

- Heat processing reduces the oxygen found in fresh food – oxygen we need to resist disease. Many physicians claim that cancer and AIDS-causing viruses thrive in blood with low oxygen levels and in the cells of people not in good health. Fresh foods contain hydrogen peroxide, which provides oxygen to kill these viruses.

- Eating heat-processed food triggers leukocytosis, a massive release of white blood cells by the body. A similar response occurs when we have an infection or are poisoned. Fresh, uncooked foods, however, do not cause such a reaction. While there is no consensus on exactly why this happens, it's clearly not a natural reaction. If the immune system is continually preoccupied with fighting off the harmful effects of consuming cooked and processed foods, its capacity to sustain optimal health is greatly reduced.

Finally, please understand that Brenda's life-changing theory, testimonials and results contained in this Living Foods Lifestyle are truly backed by more than 70 years of scientific research:

- Dr. Francis M. Pottinger's nutritional studies show that a regular diet of cooked or canned food causes the development of chronic degenerative diseases and premature mortality. He demonstrated that cooking and processing food destroys naturally occurring food enzymes. The destruction of enzymes is directly proportional to the amount of heat and processing applied to foods. Eating enzyme-depleted foods leads to the development of chronic, degenerative diseases.

  The body must expend great amounts of energy producing increased digestive enzymes to compensate for food enzymes destroyed by cooking and processing. Eating cooked foods depletes the body's "enzyme potential" and robs the body of energy needed for growth, maintenance and repair in all of its tissues and organ systems.

- Dr. Edward Howell's research prove that a diet of cooked foods causes rapid, premature mortality in mice, and that the speed of premature death is directly connected to the level of cooking temperature.

  Dr. Howell's studies show the body has a genetically determined, finite enzyme potential that is gradually depleted throughout the aging process. For example, a youth of 18 may produce amylase levels 30 times greater than those of an 85-year-old. The rate of enzyme depletion in the body is a determining factor in longevity. Enzyme-depleted foods rob the body of its enzyme potential and reduce lifespan.

- Dr. Paul Kautchakoff shows that eating cooked or processed foods causes digestive leukocytosis. Eating raw foods does not produce this reaction. The amount of digestive leukocytosis that results is directly proportional to the degree to which food has been cooked, refined, processed or manufactured.

Digestive leukocytosis is caused by "intestinal leakage," as undigested food particles leak into and attack the circulatory and lymphatic systems, becoming allergenic and toxic invaders.

In defending the body against attack by enzyme-depleted foods, the white blood cells waste their own essential enzymes and energy. This impairs the immune system's ability to defend itself against other insults, such as viruses and bacteria.

Scientific research is filled with proof that cooked and processed foods cause in humans (and animals): enzyme depletion, intestinal toxemia, auto-intoxication, constipation, leukocytosis, vitamin and mineral deficiencies, poor digestion, and assimilation and oxygen depletion.

Thanks to Brenda Cobb for presenting **The Living Foods Lifestyle** as she leads the way with her intensity and propensity for training people to dramatically heal themselves and improve their health and life.

William E. Richardson, M.D.
President and Medical Director
Atlanta Clinic of Preventive Medicine, Inc.
Atlanta, Georgia

PREFACE

I'm excited about writing this book because I'm alive and well, and the Living Foods Lifestyle is the reason. It changed my life completely. Before discovering it I was out of control and unhealthy. Now I am relaxed, in control and in perfect health, and I want to tell everyone about this Lifestyle. I am fortunate to be doing something I love with a passion, and I feel privileged to teach this life-changing Lifestyle to others. The people it brings into my life continually enrich me, and I feel it is my responsibility to teach the Living Foods Lifestyle to others in hopes that it will help them heal too. If I hadn't discovered the Lifestyle and made the changes I needed to, I might not be alive today. Teaching this information to others is my way of giving back to the world and helping to bring peace to the planet.

I'm not a doctor, nurse, certified nutritionist or dietitian. I'm just a woman telling her story of healing. I'm not trying to give anyone advice about their own health – we each must make the decisions that involve or affect our personal health. I'm just sharing information that helped me, and telling my personal story about what led me down this path. If it inspires you in some way or helps you make the changes necessary to heal, then I'm grateful.

I have never made any claims of healing others because I believe God and each individual work together to bring about healing. I don't heal anyone. I teach the principles of good health and invite those who will to join me on this wonderful journey.

I have never made any claims that this Lifestyle is for everyone or that it absolutely works for every person every time. Healing is an individual thing that encompasses the whole body, as well as the mind and the spirit. If you are on your healing journey, gather as much information about different healing modalities as you can, and then make your own decision as to what is best for you. Listen to your own inner voice.

During my healing process I realized God had a mission for me – to teach the Living Foods Lifestyle. I felt God was directing every step I took. My husband Ken, my son Richard and I were in a different field. We owned a production company and recording studio. We didn't know anything about running a Living Foods Institute. When I told them I felt we should sell the business and open a Living Foods Center, they supported me 100 percent. That has made all the difference in the world. I'm grateful to both of these wonderful men for loving me and standing by me.

People have asked how we knew what to do in the beginning, considering we'd never done this kind of work before. Our answer is that we stepped out on faith and let God guide us. We learned as we went, and we continue learning each and every day. We were fortunate to have a strong business background and we knew how to run a successful enterprise. We believe it's important to offer professional services, and we stand behind our program and our students.

As we've grown, we have remained true to one goal: building the kind of business we want to be associated with – one we can be proud to put our names on. We frequently ask ourselves, "What would I want from the program if I were a student?" We ask each student to critique the program after the session so we can improve. Our students have helped us with their ideas and suggestions, and we love them all for it. It's evident that our students love the Center, and us, because month after month they return to volunteer. They reinforce – to us and to the world – the belief that our program has changed their lives and is worth even more than they invested. More than 75 percent of our students are referred by others who experienced results after taking our program. Nothing speaks as well as satisfied clients. We are privileged to be able to help so many.

I want to acknowledge my son Rich for all of the time and effort he's put into helping me build the Living Foods Institute. In the beginning he found the perfect place for the Institute and set up all the business practices and financial programs. He managed the day-to-day business so I would be free to spread the word by teaching seminars and classes. The Institute couldn't have been so successful so quickly if not for Rich's dedication and hard work. Now another wonderful thing has come from building the Living Foods Institute: Rich has realized his true passion – working to build financial organizations. He's put tremendous effort into establishing the Institute's financial health, and now he's decided to branch out on his own helping others to establish financial health. And though we will miss him, I'm proud of him and happy that he has found his mission, as I have found mine. I speak for everyone at the Living Foods Institute when I say, "Rich, we wish you much success and happiness in all you do. Thank you for all you have done for us. We will never forget you and the love and help you have given us."

My husband Ken built the Living Foods Institute. He hammered every nail and painted every wall. A part of his wonderful energy has always been in our Center. Through his "Mr. Fix-It" business he installed reverse osmosis water filtration systems for many students and helped others with home or office repair and build-out. Every time we had a leaky faucet at the Center or needed another shelf installed or a ceiling fan hung, Ken has been there. Now that Rich has decided to pursue his dreams, Ken is joining me full time in partnership to continue to build our Institute into the most well-respected healing center for the Living Foods Lifestyle in the world. God has prepared us well with our previous experience in working together and building a successful business. Ken's devotion to me and to the health of the Living Foods Institute is evident, and our relationship gives me the strength and support I need to continue spreading the word about good health through Living Foods. Ken is a graduate of the Living Foods Institute – he completed the 10-Day Training in February 2002. The experience has made a tremendous difference in his health and his energy. He's getting younger and better looking every day!

I wrote this book to tell my personal story and to serve as an introduction to the Living Foods Lifestyle. It is by no means a complete guide, but an overview of what the Lifestyle is and how it worked for me. I hope it will get you thinking – possibly in an entirely new way. If it helps you or someone you know have the courage to step out in faith and make the changes needed to heal – even if it means going against mainstream beliefs – then I have accomplished something positive. I'm opening my heart and soul to you and telling you some really personal things. Some of these things I've never openly admitted to anyone. I'm sharing these intimate details in the hope they will help another person – perhaps someone facing a health crisis – to be strong and listen to their own inner voice for the answers.

My inner voice spoke to me loud and clear when I went to the doctor in February 1999. When he told me I had a lump in my breast and a clump of tumors on my cervix, I was scared. He sent me to the hospital so he could run tests on me and take pictures of the tumors. He told me that with my family history of breast and cervical cancer, the prognosis wasn't good. Even before tests were done he recommended immediate surgery. He said I'd better be glad that I'd come in for a checkup when I did, because it could have just saved my life.

After spending two days at the hospital and getting one test after another, the next step was to have surgery. This all happened within three or four days. It was so fast, and I felt totally overwhelmed and frightened by my doctors. They wanted me to sign a surgical consent form. They said they'd have to operate to see how extensive the tumors were. Then they'd decide if they should remove one or both breasts and do a full or partial hysterectomy. They said that after surgery, they would determine the chemotherapy and/or radiation I needed to ensure they got rid of all the cancer cells. This really scared me because I feared the worst.

I wouldn't let the doctors operate on me, so I never got absolute confirmation that I had cancer. But in my heart I knew the truth. I was the perfect candidate with my high stress, unhealthy lifestyle, and I had a high family incidence of the same type of cancers. With my new thinking and understanding of health and disease, I now realize I created my own health challenges and that it had nothing to do with what happened to other family members. Many times that can be an excuse to not face the truth: We have no one to blame for our illnesses except ourselves.

Rather than signing my life away to the doctors, I decided to find out how to heal my body naturally. I figured the odds were against me not having cancer. My mother and aunts had it, so I probably did too. As I mentioned earlier, I think differently now, and I know the disease had nothing to do with relatives. It was mine to own and take responsibility for. I remember when my mother had surgery for breast cancer (a small lump). The doctors told her they'd remove only as much breast tissue as they felt was needed. When she woke up she had no breast or lymph nodes.

I wasn't prepared to turn over my body to surgeons who seemed all too eager to cut out my body parts. I wasn't willing to give consent to them to take as much or little of my body as they deemed necessary. I wasn't willing to turn over my body and my life to people I didn't really know or trust to make the best decision for me. So, I assumed the worst, which is also what the doctors did (as they tried to scare the life out of me). Even though I didn't have the biopsies to determine if my tumors were malignant, I knew in my heart that they were, so I decided surgery and drugs wouldn't help me. I based this decision on what I had seen surgery and drugs do for other women I knew who had cancer. I saw their cancers return and even get worse after surgery and drugs. Two of my aunts died from breast and/or cervical cancer even though they had surgery and drugs more than once. They put their trust in doctors and where did it get them?

Please don't misunderstand me, I'm not suggesting other people not get biopsies, have surgery or take drugs. I realize it isn't my place to tell others what to do. I knew in my own heart and mind that these treatments weren't right for me. I'm not a doctor or healthcare professional, and I absolutely do not advise others what to do. I'm only sharing my own story and feelings, and the decisions I made for myself. I believe too many of us have given up our rights too many times, especially when it comes to our health. I believe there are too many doctors willing to cut out body parts and too many drugs being prescribed to "heal." I believe DRUGS DO NOT HEAL! I believe they are poisonous and toxic to the body. I don't believe that by destroying the body you can heal the body. That just doesn't make sense.

Why didn't I have biopsies for absolute confirmation of cancer? I decided that even if I had numbers and charts and markers of my condition, it wouldn't make any difference. I knew my body was out of balance. I knew the tumors, depression, allergies and obesity were signs that I was out of control. I'm glad I made the decision I did. And it paid off – my tumors disappeared and all the other problems resolved themselves. The body can heal itself if given the right medicine – raw and Living Foods. I only had to open my mind and heart to the possibilities.

I hope you will open your heart and mind to this information, and see if this Lifestyle feels right for you. It's up to each of us to learn and grow on our own personal journey. What you decide to do with this information is your choice. My responsibility is to tell you I believe this Lifestyle can bring health, happiness and joy to anyone who pursues it. It has certainly worked for me, and I'm grateful.

Each of you has different reasons for reading this book. Maybe it was a gift. Maybe you've heard about Living Foods and you're curious. You may have a serious health challenge, want to prevent health problems or simply maintain the health you have now. Maybe you want to help someone you care about. Whatever your reason for reading this book, I hope you find the information you seek. Further, I hope you'll be encouraged to try the Living Foods Lifestyle and see what it can do for you. You'll never know how great it is until you actually experience the benefits for yourself.

I can't take credit for this incredible Lifestyle – my teachings are based on those of Ann Wigmore. I learned about the Living Foods Lifestyle by visiting the Ann Wigmore Foundation in New Mexico and by reading every one of Wigmore's books I could get my hands on. I feel the information in those books is priceless and must be imparted to future generations. I am only a messenger passing on the brilliant teachings of others before me. I give complete credit to Ann Wigmore for all information about the Living Foods Lifestyle in this book. I learned from her books, and now I've put her teachings into my own words. It's my way of carrying on her work and her important message of healing.

I never had the privilege of meeting Ann Wigmore; she died in a fire at her Boston Institute years before I discovered the Living Foods Lifestyle. However, I have great respect for this remarkable woman who developed the Lifestyle I credit with saving my life. She lived the Lifestyle for more than 35 years, setting an excellent example for all of us to follow. I make every effort to stay as true as possible to Wigmore's original teachings. She developed and taught this information to thousands of people, and I believe she knew what she was talking about. It worked well then, and it continues to help many more today. It's ageless and timeless – the original way humans ate. There's no reason to change it, because it works beautifully just the way it is. I love the simplicity of it, and the ease with which you can put it to work in your life, no matter where you live.

I honor Ann Wigmore every day for the healing energy and love she put into her work. I've done my best to practice the Living Foods Lifestyle since first learning about it in February 1999 and I will, to the best of my ability, share Wigmore's information about the Living Foods Lifestyle with others who want to live a healthy, disease-free life.

As my knowledge of raw and Living Foods has grown and expanded, I have also been influenced by such authors as Viktoras Kulvinskas (*Survival Into The 21st Century*); David Wolfe (*The Sunfood Diet Success System*); and Dr. Norman Walker (*Colon Health*). In this book, I'm sharing with you what others have taught me and what I now teach to my own students.

This information is neither new nor new age – this idea and way of living have been around for centuries. It's the way man lived and ate long before the discovery of fire. I've added gourmet recipes to the basic Living Foods Lifestyle, to keep people interested and to help them make the transition from eating a cooked food diet. But the truth is that simpler is better. The longer I continue in this Lifestyle, the simpler I eat. In the beginning I ate the gourmet recipes, but as time passes, I find a piece of fruit, some sprouts, greens or a simple vegetable satisfies me. I don't need fancy dishes anymore. However, they were a great help when I was first making the transition from cooked food.

That's an important lesson I've learned, and which I impart to you: Keep things easy and fun – enjoy your journey to better health and a better life. This Lifestyle isn't complicated or overwhelming. Like anything new, it may take a little adjusting and some re-thinking of old ideas, but pretty soon you'll feel as though you've done it forever. And the longer you do it, the easier it gets. This Lifestyle can save you time and money while restoring you to perfect health. Just relax and let go of any preconceived notions. The only way to know if it's right for you is to try it. Then and only then will you see the results you long for – total health, vibrant energy and a sense of complete well-being. Make no judgments until you have actually done it.

When I developed the Living Foods Institute's detoxification and rebuilding program I decided it should last 10 consecutive days. This was different from other raw and Living Foods programs I was familiar with that ran for 14 to 28 days. I knew God, with Divine Intelligence, was at work in all my decisions. I listened to my inner voice as God told me what to do.

I didn't really realize just how profound a decision it was to run the program for 10 days instead of 12, 14 or 20. Until, that is, one of my students came to day seven of her class and said, "I brought you something from the Bible that says exactly what you're doing here, and it reminds me of you and your staff. You folks are living this scripture." When I read the passage, it blew me away. I grew up in the Baptist church and I knew of this scripture, but over the years I'd forgotten it. I believe God has a Divine Plan and all of us are part of it. God sends us messages all the time to confirm that we are doing the right thing. In fact, I'm constantly reminded that the work I'm doing is indeed God's work. When I read this scripture it was another reminder that I'm living my mission in life. I'd like to share this passage with you:

> *Daniel resolved not to defile himself with the royal food and wine, and he asked the chief official for permission not to defile himself this way. Now God had caused the official to show favor and sympathy to Daniel, but the official told Daniel, "I am afraid of my lord the king, who has assigned your food and drink. Why should he see you looking worse than the other young men your age? The king would then have my head because of you."*

> *Daniel then said to the guard whom the chief official had appointed over Daniel, "Please test your servants for 10 days: Give me nothing but vegetables to eat and water to drink. Then compare my appearance with that of the young men who eat the royal food, and treat your servants in accordance with what you see." So he agreed to this and tested him for 10 days.*

> *At the end of 10 days he looked healthier and better nourished than any of the young men who ate the royal food. So the guard took away their choice food and the wine they were to drink and gave them vegetables instead.*

> *To Daniel God gave knowledge and understanding of all kinds of literature and learning. And Daniel could understand visions and dreams of all kinds.*

> *At the end of the time set by the king to bring Daniel in, the chief official presented him to Nebuchadnezzar. The king talked with*

him, and he found none equal to Daniel: so he entered the king's service. In every matter of wisdom and understanding about which the king questioned Daniel, he found him 10 times better than all the magicians and enchanters in his whole kingdom.

Daniel 1:8-20

Nothing happens by accident. The way I planned the 10-day training wasn't an accident. It's no accident that you're reading this book. The timing is right, and you're ready to hear the information. You're ready for exciting news about an incredible Lifestyle that can give you total and perfect health – body, mind, and spirit. You're ready to reclaim your power. You've probably heard the saying, "When the student is ready, the teacher will appear." That's exactly how I felt when I found out about the Living Foods Lifestyle, and maybe that's how you feel too. At the time in my life when I needed it most, it made itself known to me.

I was an eager student, ready to learn all I could. At the same time, I feared the changes I had to make. My advice to you is to relax and enjoy the learning process. Focus less on the destination so you can enjoy the journey. Don't worry about what you don't know, or the changes you'll be making. Don't get caught up in the details. "Be still and know" that this is "the way, the truth, and the light." Embrace the opportunity to learn and grow in a positive way. You can make a transition from a poor lifestyle to a healthy one with ease, happiness and joy. Don't be afraid to embrace new ideas and new thoughts. They can make a difference not only in how you feel, but also in the true state of your health – body, mind and spirit. No matter how hard it is to step out of your comfort zone, step on out anyway. Don't hold back. You're ready, and we're here to help.

I tell students when they come to the Institute to take the 10-Day Program that they shouldn't make any judgments until they have completed the 10 days. We cover a lot of material in those 10 days, and to some of our students, it's quite radical. I remind everyone that if they don't want to take all they learn with them, they can leave any part they choose behind. Keeping an open mind, not judging and embracing new ideas is important when you embark on this Lifestyle. No one will "make" you do this program. No one will insist that you become a 100 percent raw and Living Foodist. Just get started, whether it's 10 percent, 50 percent or 70 percent, or any amount you choose. Begin today and just take one day at a time. Who knows, maybe you'll feel better than you've ever felt, and one day you'll want to become a 100 percent raw and Living Foodist – not because I say so, but because you feel the difference. It's all up to you!

Don't take my word for it. The only way you'll ever know if this will work for you is to do it yourself. Then you can make your own judgments. Have fun on your journey and enjoy each and every experience. Get as much out of life as you possibly can and always give UNCONDITIONAL LOVE!

I am excited to tell you that since the first printing of this book, we have now expanded the Living Foods Institute to reach an international audience. We are currently holding our 10-Day Course in both Atlanta, Georgia, and Miami Beach, Florida. No matter which location you choose, you will receive the best possible training in the Living Foods Lifestyle offered anywhere in the world. We remain true to the original teachings of Dr. Ann Wigmore. Thousands have now heard our message and have experienced their own personal healings. I hope you will join us in one of our 10-Day Trainings and find out just what we can do for you.

B.C.

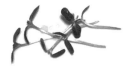

TESTIMONIALS

Before I tell my story, I want to share testimonials from Living Foods Institute staff and students. Realize that no matter how sick you are today, you can restore your health. Not only did it work for me, it has worked for many others. For more testimonials, visit our Web site, www.livingfoodsinstitute.com.

The success of the Living Foods Institute is due to the loving and caring teaching staff who help me teach the 10-Day Program and give ongoing support and encouragement to our students. They give their all to help heal the world one person at a time.

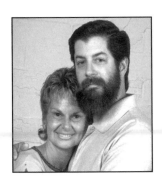

KEN COBB
I am so glad my wife chose to heal herself the natural way. It has completely changed her life and mine, too.

I have been a meat and fast-food eater and beer drinker for many years. Quite frankly I never even gave that much thought to my diet.

Then I watched how Brenda changed so

1

dramatically when she adopted the Living Foods Lifestyle. Some of it even rubbed off on me and in February 2002, I took the 10-Day Living Foods Lifestyle course myself. I lost weight and my blood pressure went down.

I found out during the program that my cholesterol was high and that I needed to do something about it. I drink wheatgrass juice and Rejuvelac every day, no more beer. I don't eat as much meat and dairy as I once did. Now I eat a veggie burger when I want cooked food. I still eat some cooked food, but I eat more raw and Living Foods now than I ever have. My cholesterol has dropped into the normal ranges and I have more energy and feel better than I have in years.

Even if you don't intend to go 100 percent raw and Living Foods you can still get some great results. I'm proof of that. I enjoy working with Brenda at the Center and helping her spread the word about the Living Foods Lifestyle.

I used to own my own "Mr. Fix-it" business, but closed that business and joined Brenda full-time to support her in fulfilling her Divine Mission. I'm so glad I did.

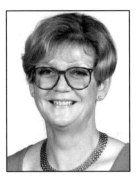

ANN HALLEWELL

My journey to the Living Foods Institute began before the Institute was ever conceived!

In the late 1990s I was looking for alternative ways to deal with menopausal symptoms and my own "personal summers" (hot flashes). I went to a seminar in my local aesthetician's office titled *"How To Treat Menopause Naturally."* By the end of the seminar I knew I'd been "taken by the hand" by a power far greater than anything else I knew, and I was going on a journey to help heal the world.

Always an avid reader, I was reading books on how our environment, diet, thought patterns and spirituality affect our overall health. I contacted Trinity College of Natural Health, and completed the classwork to become a Natural Health Professional

I'm now following Trinity's program to become a doctor of naturopathy.

I attended a seminar hosted by Brenda Cobb and Richard Byrd on January 31, 2000. Everything I'd been learning on my journey of alternative health and natural medicine was endorsed that evening. The body innately knows how to heal itself, given the right nourishment and health regime. Death begins in the colon, cooking foods destroys the valuable enzymes and you should eat a predominately raw diet.

I knew I was going to take the 10-Day Program at The Living Foods Institute and I did, completing the course April 16, 2000. Those 10 days changed my life completely!

When I entered the Center April 7, I weighed 210 pounds. I lost 11 pounds during the 10-Day Program. I now weigh 150 pounds. I effortlessly lost 60 pounds, and my weight is still reducing.

My "personal summers" are a thing of the past, I require less sleep, mild depression has gone and I enjoy a wonderful feeling when walking – it feels as though my feet never touch the ground. In addition to this, I've noticed a huge shift in my mindset – nothing ever seems to be insurmountable. It really is incredible!

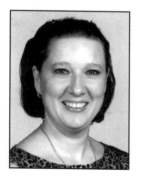

JOANNE TRINH

I first heard of the Living Foods Institute in June 2000. I'd been searching for a diet or lifestyle change that would fit with vegetarianism – it seemed so many diets required a lot of meat and dairy products. When I heard about the Living Foods Lifestyle, it was the first time a diet made real sense to me.

I came to the Center in July 2000 not because of a health crisis, but for weight loss. At the time I weighed more than 165 pounds. I'm not sure how much more, because I refused to weigh myself after I reached that point.

During the 10-Day Program I lost 18 pounds. I did three enemas a day and three colonics during the first 10 days of the program to get my colon cleaned out. It was unheard of for me to lose weight so easily. I'd been doing aerobic exercises for years, barely losing a pound or two a week and then gaining it right back, plus some.

I was frustrated at the time because I'd always been interested in health and nutrition. I was a vegetarian for 13 years, thinking that was the best I could do, but still wondering why I was overweight. My husband, who is Oriental, weighs only 98 pounds. When we got married I weighed only 95 pounds, so being overweight was hard for me to accept.

One of the reasons I'm a vegetarian is because I'm also a Christian. I live my life based on Genesis 1:29, which says that God has told us to eat for our food seed-bearing fruit, herbs, greens and vegetables.

It never dawned on me that in the beginning food was never cooked and fire was not yet discovered. God knew just what he was doing when he put raw, Living Foods on the earth with just the right amount of enzymes, vitamins and minerals. Who was I to alter this perfect diet in any way? Eat it the way God gave it to us – not cooked!

Six months before I came to the Center, my pastor asked our congregation this question: "Why did God put you here?" We had to write the answer down and provide a picture so he and the rest of the congregation could pray over it.

As I prayed over the paper, the first thing I wrote was that I wanted to teach people about health and nutrition. I looked at what I had written and asked myself, "How can I do this when I am so overweight myself? Who would ever listen to me?"

It took me only four to six months to lose 50 to 60 pounds. I went from a size 13-14 to a size 5-6; from more than 165 pounds to between 105 and 110 pounds. I no longer have acid reflux or shortness of breath. I sleep less now, only four to six hours rather than eight to 10 hours. Three days into the 10-Day Program, I knew this is where "God wanted me to be."

I asked Brenda if I could work for her and I started August 8, 2000. I know this is my calling. Everything comes naturally and it feels good to be helping other people heal their lives one day at a time. It is truly a blessing to me, sent from God.

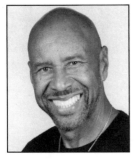

REED EVANS-WRIGHT

During the mid-1990s I was plagued with multiple health problems. I'd had full-blown asthma since 1994, high blood pressure (174/114), allergies and abnormal blood sugar levels. During my struggle with these conditions, I believed I ate fairly well and always exercised. I chose not to do conventional medical treatments for these challenges; I knew there had to be a better way.

A friend introduced me to the the Living Foods Lifestyle. On March 18, 2000, I went to the Annapurna Retreat in Port Townsend, Washington, on a full-time quest. I stayed for a full week, and during this time I experienced many profound changes.

After three days on the Lifestyle, my blood pressure went down to 117/77. Along with the program, I received three colonics and my weight dropped 23 pounds. After 90 days on the program, my weight went from 210 pounds to 150 pounds, where it has now stabilized. My asthma was completely gone in 90 days, and my allergies cleared up.

After leaving the retreat, I returned to Olympia, Washington, where I lived. I looked for a raw foods community for support, but I was unable to find one. Traveling on Easter holiday to Atlanta, Georgia, I was shocked and pleased to find an article written by Brenda Cobb in *Aquarius* magazine about the raw and Living Foods Lifestyle. They may have been Brenda's words, but they were my sentiments. After contacting her, I was soon enrolled in the program.

The real test for me came in July 2001. I broke my femur in a serious fall, requiring extensive surgery and nearly two weeks' hospitalization. At the end of those two weeks, I left the hospital on crutches and resumed my teaching responsibilities.

Much to my doctors' surprise, by four weeks postoperative my break was nearly healed. Through this entire hospitalization and recovery, I remained 100 percent faithful to the program with Living Foods, colonics and enemas, massage and a positive attitude. I am convinced I owe my recovery to the dramatic changes I've embraced in my life.

I've been convinced for the last 20 years that all human

misery is the result of ignorance, and nothing but knowledge will free us from this ignorance and its effects. The knowledge I am talking about is knowledge of self – especially the knowledge of what to feed oneself.

LONG-TERM PRESCRIPTION DRUG USE / CANDIDA AND SYSTEMIC YEAST INFECTION

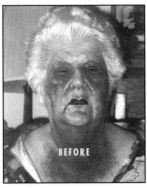

BEFORE

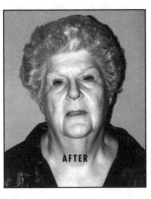

AFTER

DOLORES REAVIS Atlanta, Georgia
My name is Dolores and I'm 76 years old. My health problems began in my late 20s when I was diagnosed with a thyroid problem. My body didn't tolerate the medications I was given. Upon seeing a new doctor, I was given a prescription for Dexedrine (diet pills). This was the beginning of my drug addiction.

I've been married three times and have four children. With my first pregnancy I suffered from nausea, hypertension, toxemia, convulsions and albumin in my urine. The process was the same for the other three pregnancies, with the exception of convulsions. Each labor was long and difficult. Despite this I was always back at work a week to 10 days after each delivery.

By age 31, my fourth child was born and I was taking Dexedrine, full-strength Phenobarbital and Codeine. Six months later I had hepatitis, jaundice and gallstones. I had my gallbladder removed and was back at work within 10 days. I had a thriving beauty salon where I'd worked for 18 to 20 hours a day for 20 years doing show work, platform work, TV work and fantasy shows with models.

In my early 40s, I checked myself into Battle Creek Mental Health Unit where my sister was a nurse. I stayed for a month and spent the majority of it asleep. What I learned was that after having four children and working all those hours and years, I'd used up all my energy by being Superwoman. The doctors never mentioned I was a prescription drug addict.

At 42 I contracted viral pneumonia and was hospitalized. I was given 13 shots of antibiotics in 30 hours. It wasn't until six weeks later that I realized some of these shots had hit my sciatic nerve. I'd partially lost the use of my right hand, and I was dragging my right foot, experiencing horrendous pain. My chiropractor worked hard over a long period of time to eliminate the pain and was able to restore the use of my hand and my foot within eight weeks.

At 52, realizing I had a problem, I started Al-Anon. It was there I met my sponsor, Joy Sedgeman, to whom I will be eternally grateful. I divorced my third husband, who was an alcoholic, so I could concentrate on healing myself. It was only after four years of Al-Anon that I realized that for the past 25 years I'd had a prescription drug addiction. Between the ages of 30 and 52 I saw psychiatrists, psychologists and therapists. All they ever told me was that I was a "hard worker, very talented and an over-achiever." I dealt with the pain, tears and fears through daily meetings and retreats.

Because I was physically ill, mentally disturbed, emotionally empty, spiritually bankrupt and hardly able to function at any level, I attracted unstable, addictive partners. My weight gain began at age 55. By 64 my body was like raw hamburger meat from my chest up to my forehead. I was grotesque … open running sores, my eyes were swollen nearly shut, and I had an elevated temperature. About four times a year I would break out in the Candida, which would overtake my body.

In November 2000, my chiropractor, who kept me alive with food supplements and chiropractic care, suggested I go to a clinical laboratory for a full spectrum of blood tests. The results said my gut was in the worst possible condition and about to shut down. The toxins and poisons in my body were at a level of grave concern.

By the beginning of 2001 I knew I was fading fast. I'd had so many chemical burnoffs caused by Candida that I knew I had to try something new. I saw Dr. William Richardson at the Atlanta Clinic of Preventive Medicine. He confirmed that my body was full of Candida.

After going through detox programs with Dr. Richardson, it was suggested that I come to the Living Foods Institute. I took the September 2001 class and felt well enough to become a volunteer at the November 10-Day Training. When I walked into the Center each day, the staff members would say, "WOW" as they saw my much improved and partially healed skin and open eyes. At this point I have lost 60 pounds and am still detoxing – not only physically but also emotionally.

If I eat fruit, specifically and most dangerously citrus, I will become totally and uncontrollably intoxicated. At this point in time I am eating only the four healing foods and expect to have to remain on them for some time to come.

I still have a way to go, but you can see from the before and after pictures that I am on my way to much better health. I thank Brenda Cobb and her staff for all their help, support, love and their hugs.

PROSTATE CANCER

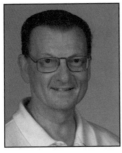

GENE LOWE Acworth, Georgia

In June 1999 I was diagnosed with prostate cancer. I saw three urologists and one radiologist. The urologists wanted to remove my prostate along with the tumor. The radiologist wanted to implant radioactive seeds, then "shoot" me with external radiation to kill both the prostate and the tumor. During the time it took to visit all these doctors, I was introduced to alternative treatments ranging from fermented soybean extract to proven herbs that would shrink the tumor and, I hoped, kill the cancer cells. I chose this program rather than what the doctors prescribed.

During this treatment, a friend who'd heard Brenda Cobb speak at a seminar introduced me to the Living Foods Institute. I knew right away this was the "missing link" between Chinese herbs and complete healing. I enrolled in the course immediately, attended the class and have been eating natural foods now for about seven months. My PSA (Prostate Specific Antigen – a test that shows toxins and bacteria in the blood) count had risen to a high of 11.2. Anything above 4 is suspicious; anything above 6 is most likely prostate cancer. Two months ago, it was down to 4.4. I give all the credit to the application of what I learned at the school, to wheatgrass implants and supplements I continue to take. Without this course, I am sure I would not be able to write this letter. But with it, I will be around for a long time. I thank God I found an answer that the entire world should know.

UTERINE / CERVICAL CANCER

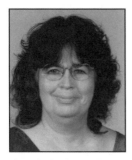

MARCIA JONES Marietta, Georgia

In February 1979, after months of terrible periods, funky discharge and then Stage III, IV, and V pap smears, a GYN at Stanford University looked me in the eye and said: "If you don't have a hysterectomy within two months, you'll be dead in six months."

I looked him right back in the eye, said, "I don't think so," and walked out of his office. I firmly believed God sent me down to this planet with those parts, and that I would leave the planet with those parts. More than that, I didn't feel that my time on Earth was through. My son was about to be 12 years old, and deep inside I knew I would see him grow up.

Uterine and cervical cancer are technically two different types of cancer, and both were Stage IV. The only medical procedure I allowed was cryotherapy – freezing the inner lining of the uterus, which then necrotizes and sheds. I did this three times. The doctors at Stanford were furious and said I'd be dead in six months. That was 1979. Well, I'm not dead and I had no surgery, no chemotherapy and no radiation.

What I did was look at other species on the planet. I looked at their diets and realized they didn't alter their food. They didn't process it and they didn't cook it. And no other species took in dairy products (from their own or other species) after weaning.

I began sprouting my own sprouts – you couldn't get them in stores then. I made Rejuvelac – I'd heard about Ann Wigmore's program in 1974 and had made and enjoyed it even before my diagnosis. I took in lots of wheatgrass and juiced, juiced, juiced! I had a 20' x 70' organic garden that I tended, as did residents of all five houses in our California commune. I went out in the garden and "grazed." I did eat brown rice at the time, but I realize now that digesting the rice slowed my recovery. It didn't stop it, just slowed it down.

We know a lot more now and people are doing in three months what it took me more than a year to do "hit and miss." I took

Brenda's class to gain some of this "new" knowledge and to get to know more people in this Lifestyle. I'm glad I did. As founder and international director of The Dixie PMS & Menopause Center (www.tidesoflife.com) I encounter many women who have "gotten off track" healthwise, and for whom Brenda's class could be – if nothing else – the greatest anti-aging program currently available.

To anyone out there who has issues with energy, stamina, etc., or who has an actual "disease" condition such as cancer, diabetes or just about anything else, this is what I would say: DO YOURSELF A FAVOR! If you're ready to take responsibility for your health and get your health back, investigate this program. Come to Atlanta and take the 10-day immersion program which jump-starts the process. Brenda knows what she's doing and she has the most current knowledge available to give you. Her own life is a Living Foods testimonial you can trust.

HIV / AIDS

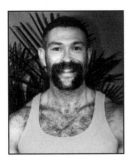

CRAIG DOYLE Atlanta, Georgia
Living Foods has definitely changed my life for the better! I was diagnosed with HIV in February 1990. My lover, who was tested at the same time, died nine months later. During the next years, I took many medications and therapies. I tried different alternative, holistic and metaphysical combinations. Some helped but didn't provide the key. Many physicians, practitioners and healers offered perspectives and insights, but my immune system continued to decline. My physician prescribed several anti-virals; they seemed to work for a while, but eventually failed. I found I'd used all the medications – some approved, some not approved. I experienced much anger and resentment. What I was really feeling was fear – fear that my options were coming to an end.

Miraculously, I was introduced to Brenda Cobb. I told her about my situation and desire to change. She could see how I looked and felt. She said she was going to bring me some Energy Soup the next day, and asked me if I'd try it. I told her I'd try anything at this point. The next day she brought me a quart jar of this green "goop." I said I couldn't drink that; it would make me throw up. She reminded me that I wanted a change and that I said I'd try anything. So I tried it. It was green, yes, but I thought it was pretty tasty. She brought me a quart of soup every day for several weeks. I started really liking it. The soup helped me to begin detoxing, but I'm not one to quit because of little speed bumps.

My perseverance paid off. After several days, people who I had never spoken to began to approach me about what I was doing. They commented on how good I looked. Some said I had a spark in my eye, and noted how clear my skin appeared. I noticed I didn't need as much sleep. My energy increased and I didn't need to nap in the middle of the day. I could see a marked improvement in several weeks. My friends and associates thought I was crazy. Everyone had something to say about my Energy Soup. Curiosity was rampant. Some people even became angry. I realized that was their fear and doubt surfacing. Most people, however, were inquisitive. They want-ed more information.

Then came a true test. My blood tests showed that my body liked what it was getting. My liver tests showed improvement, my blood counts increased and my T-cell counts increased. All the nurs-es and my doctor talked about how well I looked. They were surprised when I told them what I was doing.

Since I met Brenda my life has improved and my perspectives have changed. I rid myself of "poisonous" relationships. I saw how I'd been holding myself from growth and personal power. My awareness of spirit has developed and clarified. My family, friends and those people I see and say hello to have spoken on how much joy and hap-piness I seem to be feeling. I am go glad I took the Living Foods Lifestyle course with Brenda Cobb. I feel alive!

HIV / SINUS / RESPIRATORY ALLERGIES

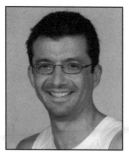

BOB BOURGEOIS Atlanta, Georgia
As a chronic sufferer of sinus and respiratory allergies, intestinal irregularities and fatigue (to the point that I'd fall asleep at my desk), I spent years going to doctors and specialists trying to evaluate my symptoms. I often wondered if my health conditions were a result of the numerous rounds of antibiotics I took in my adolescence

and young adulthood, first to combat acne, and then later, the recurring sinus and throat infections my allergies would bring on. In the 12 years I searched for relief, I experienced marginal symptom reduction through the use of various prescription drugs. I never obtained full relief though, and was uncomfortable with putting chemicals into my body, especially when they were not producing acceptable results. I knew inside there had to be a better way.

Then, in January 2000, my world turned upside down. I started off the new century diagnosed with an HIV infection. After the initial wave of emotions passed, I instinctively knew that adhering to the prescribed treatment regime – filling my body with highly toxic chemicals to fight the virus and contending with their numerous side effects – was not the course of action I wished to pursue. I knew within the first five minutes of hearing those words from my doctor that I needed to make my body as healthy as possible. I needed to do all I could to aid and support it in its fight against the virus. My course of action was to change my diet, exercise, mediate and take yoga classes. I was beginning a journey of getting to know, beginning to respect and beginning to love the inner me. Over the course of the next year, I watched the concentration of virus in my body (my viral load) fluctuate from low readings of 42,000 up to as high as 103,000.

After eight months of weekly visits to a Chinese acupuncturist (two to three times a week) and the lifestyle changes I had incorporated, I had a viral load reading in February 2001 of 28,300. I was pleased with the results my efforts had produced, and determined to continue helping and supporting my body as it healed itself. That's when I turned to the Living Foods Institute. This would be the next leg of my journey to health. I had attended a seminar at the Living Foods Institute in February 2000, shortly after my diagnosis, but I wasn't ready to make the commitment at that time. My life was already in so much turmoil; to churn it up further was not something I could do at that moment. I had healing I needed to do first.

A year later I was ready to listen to the message again and put its teachings into practice. I went 100 percent raw and Living Foods on March 8, 2001, and remained that way for the duration of the 10-day class. A week after class ended, I was re-tested and my viral load count had dropped from 28,300 to 10,300. My T-cells had gone up from 250 to 360. My doctor was thrilled and encouraged me to, "continue doing whatever it is you're doing."

Now my viral load reading is 3,030 and my T-cell count is 360 – quite an improvement. As an added bonus, my chronic sinus allergies and infections did not rear their ugly heads this past spring. Although I cannot say I was completely symptom-free during the height of pollen season, I can say there was a 90 percent improvement in my symptoms over previous years. There were no sinus or throat infections and my headache and respiratory discomfort was minimal. For these things I am truly amazed. On top of that, I can actually make it through an afternoon at work without wanting to close my eyes and sleep.

As I incorporate the Living Foods Lifestyle further into my daily life, I'm becoming aware of how my body responds when I eat things that are not in my best interest. I see symptoms begin to recur as I fall back into old health patterns. The allergies, fatigue and ill health all begin to return. I'm becoming acutely aware of how what I put into my body affects the way it functions. I have many years of poor living choices – and their effects on my body – to overcome and reverse. But for the first time in a long time, I see a light at the end of the tunnel. I have a ray of hope that grows stronger and stronger as I continue to repair and rebuild my health naturally. I know the body is truly an amazing, self-healing gift. When it's treated with respect and love, it can overcome any challenge. The next time you hear from me, I'll be telling you that I have been completely transformed, that I feel vibrant and alive and that HIV is no longer a part of my life. Consider joining me as I walk down this path of self-discovery, as I learn how to love and respect myself and the world around me.

WEIGHT LOSS / CANDIDA

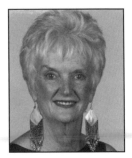

PEG SHEPHERD Marietta, Georgia
In August 2000 I called Brenda Cobb and told her that all my life I'd tried to lose weight. I'd tried every fad diet I heard about, lost and then regained even more. From December 1998 to August 2000 I had lost from 230 pounds to 190 pounds by modifying my diet, but I was stuck. My metabolism simply did not work anymore, and I really didn't believe that could be changed.

I told Brenda I had all the diets out of my system. I did not want to try any others. I asked her if she could help me. She said, "Come and see."

On August 30, 2000 I started her class. I ate only the healing foods during that time and I lost about 15 pounds. I began to feel so good! Since that time I have not eaten cooked food again, and in March 2001, I weighed 122 pounds (a weight I hadn't seen since I was 10 years old). By May, my weight had stabilized at 135 pounds, and I now wear size 6. With the Living Foods Lifestyle, I'm thankful I don't have to come off my diet and go on maintenance. I am very happy with the gracious plentiful food I daily enjoy.

Other Results:

Hair: For 30 years I colored my graying hair and it became so shocking white I had to have the roots colored every four weeks. Since taking the Living Foods Lifestyle course, I decided to leave the color off to watch the process of change. One morning I looked in the mirror and saw that it had a definitely darker cast. It has been gradual, but at the scalp you can see the darker hairs coming in. Now the white hairs are coming out by the handful. I had a haircut this week and my beautician said, "Your hair is growing like wildfire." She even had to thin it.
Facial Hair: I no longer need to have my lip and chin waxed.
Skin: Wrinkles, scar tissue and warts are going away; with exercise, loose skin from losing 108 pounds is not a problem.
Candida: In 1999 I had a Body Scan, which revealed that I had three of the 11 kinds: Candida Lusitani, Candida Rugoso and Candida Krusei. In February 2001, my re-scan showed no Candida!
Energy: I recently celebrated my 60th birthday, and now I can go up and down Kennesaw Mountain in 45 minutes, which is a record for me. Four to six hours sleep is all I need.

I now feel each meal is a feast, and I'm so glad that when people drop by, I can prepare something wonderful to share with them (at their level) within a few minutes.

At last I have learned how to eat, and I'm developing a body beyond my wildest imagination. Thank you, Brenda Cobb, what a priceless gift you have given to so many. We are blessed to have you in Atlanta.

DEPRESSION / BLOOD PRESSURE / CHOLESTEROL

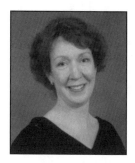

BEA YORKER San Francisco, California
Four years ago, at the age of 44, I began having what I thought were perimenopausal symptoms. My worst symptoms were panic attacks and insomnia. I was waking up at 4:00 a.m. feeling like Chicken Little thinking, "The sky is falling, the sky is falling." When I started waking at 2:00 a.m., I knew I needed help. I was also experiencing increased PMS symptoms, feeling suicidal and homicidal for several hours each month. As a nursing professor, university administrator and mother of three, I had to be able to function.

I'm a health-conscious person. I've been doing transcendental meditation twice a day for 22 years, juice fasting for 10 days at a time once a year, and I've been in psychotherapy and family therapy on and off for years. I was open to seeing a psychiatrist who prescribed Prozac.

It opened my eyes – I felt I was more the person I was meant to be, I overcame profound feelings of unworthiness I'd experienced since childhood and my sleep returned to normal. Prozac allowed me to do work in family therapy that I had previously not been able to do. I finally set limits on my husband's verbal abuse toward the children and me. I felt worthy enough to realize that my marriage was exploitative with me "bringing home the bacon, frying it up in a pan, and never letting him forget he's a man."

To make a long story short, my children were old enough that I got a divorce. All was fine until the Prozac seemed to stop working. I was convinced I had received a placebo by mistake and argued with the pharmacist, who gently told me I probably needed my dose checked.

Sure enough, my psychiatrist said this was common and I could go up to a dosage that felt right. I spent nine months on 60 milligrams (three pills) a day until my friends told me I seemed a bit manic. I reduced the dose to 40 milligrams and continued juggling medications with my psychiatrist's help. In 1999 she suggested Wellbutrin (the stop-smoking medicine, Zyban) to alleviate the side effects of Prozac; namely a 20-pound weight gain and lack of energy. It helped.

But by January 2000 I felt the medicines were giving me problems. When I had a general physical, my blood pressure was 148/104. I was stunned and felt the Wellbutrin had caused this, so I promptly stopped it. I was prescribed Ziac, a combination beta-blocker and diuretic. I felt better, but my energy and ability to think were affected. I reached a low point when I cried to my boss and said that my ability to write and publish articles as I'd been doing for 15 years was gone.

Because I'm an active healthcare consumer, I remembered an enlightened endocrinologist I worked with years ago at Emory Hospital, Dr. Harry Delcher, who fasted adult onset diabetics for two weeks before giving them medications. He was able to reverse the diabetes in about half his patients. I went to see him, and along with advising me not to seek symptom relief for issues I needed to face, he gave me low-dose estrogen and thyroid to see if my energy and thinking would improve.

After the first month of taking two Prozac, Ziac for my blood pressure, estrogen patches, and thyroid every day, AND FEELING NO BETTER, I felt that if this was as good as medicine could get me, it wasn't worth it. Then the doctor called me and told me my cholesterol was 335. I requested a three-month sick leave from my university job (I had accumulated almost five months of leave) so I could stop the medications, meditate, practice yoga and fast my blood pressure and cholesterol down.

Needless to say, this caused some controversy at the university. I believe that as a nurse, if I can't heal my own ills through lifestyle changes, I can't ask my patients to either. I found the Living Foods Institute as I began my leave. I stopped all medications cold turkey. I did detox and had some tearful days, but nothing as bad as I had feared. I have continued drinking 2 ounces of wheatgrass juice and eating Living Foods every day.

The Living Foods 10-Day Program not only allowed me to stop all five medicines I was taking, it actually may have buffered my detoxification. I could feel what was detox from sugar, caffeine, alcohol and cooked foods because I have fasted in the past. However, the healing foods, and especially the wheatgrass juice, seemed to make the sudden stoppage of medications easier. Although I had some emotional discomfort on and off for a month, my blood pressure fell to 120/84 by the end of the 10 days.

After a month of total Living Foods Lifestyle my blood pressure was 104/68 and my cholesterol came down 82 points. That is truly dramatic. The month of raw foods prepared me well for a juice fast, and then I eased back to raw foods and took up yoga to strengthen my body after the fast. I now feel that my body is manufacturing its own serotonin, endorphins, dopamine and epinephrine. I can feel my organs and glands functioning the way they are supposed to. I am still coping with depression and sad moods, but my physical state, my mental acuity and my sleep are all so vastly improved that it's worth it, and I know it will continue to gradually improve.

It has been a year since I completed the Living Foods course. I am now 48 years old, I continue yoga five times a week and I eat 80 percent raw. My blood pressure is maintained around 125/84. I am so grateful to be off the medicine and having a healthy menopause. My figure is terrific and my skin glows.

MIGRAINE HEADACHES / CHRONIC FATIGUE SYNDROME

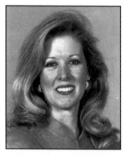

GINA E. JONES Smyrna, Georgia
I'd like to thank Brenda Cobb and the Living Foods Institute for giving me my life back! The last few years seemed to be an endless downward spiral. I was diagnosed with seemingly "unrelated" health problems such as migraines, endometriosis, chronic fatigue, PMS, fibromyalgia, allergies and leaky gut syndrome. These "challenges" were further complicated by the diagnosis of mercury and lead poisoning.

Working diligently with an environmental and preventative health doctor in Atlanta helped address some of these issues. However, the daily headaches and migraines never went away. I was living on Advil and Darvon just to get through each day. My doctor's advice was to try and find a job that was in a "less toxic" environment. I'd been a flight attendant for 23 years, and my doctor said my body had reached a toxic overload of chemicals. Being a single parent and trying to start a new job while working to heal myself was not an option. Somehow I'd have to work through these issues.

When I heard Brenda speak at a local health food store, I

finally heard the truth! Everything she said made sense. I knew the answer had to be simple, but everyone tries to make it complicated – and make money off our problems. The pharmaceutical companies want to make money from drugs, doctors want to keep us sick (great job security) by their lack of knowledge and supplement providers aren't a whole lot different from the drug corporations.

It basically comes to this…what you put in is what you get out. It's as simple as that! After learning through Brenda and the Living Foods Institute how to prepare foods, eat properly and allow my body to heal naturally, the results have been phenomenal. Since taking the class in November 2000, I haven't had a migraine or a headache. That's a miracle. And, I didn't have to quit my job.

All my PMS symptoms, which were becoming worse every month, totally disappeared during the first cycle after the class. My skin looks great and the bonus is I lost the 35 pounds that slowly crept on during the last few years. Everyone told me these conditions were normal because I was over 40. I knew they weren't. Brenda Cobb and the Living Foods Institute proved that! I now eat food that I was told to avoid and enjoy my meals without the pain and discomfort associated before.

I have energy again, look great and am healing myself through Living Foods. Once again I enjoy my life, my family and my job. Thanks, Brenda, for giving me my life back!

BLOOD PRESSURE / CHOLESTEROL

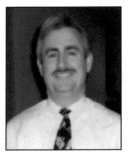

JOHN O'NEAL Atlanta, Georgia
I'm a married, 49-year-old professional male who was once called the "King of the Carnivores" by friends and family. Over the years, I'd become obese and was more than 30 pounds overweight. At my last annual physical, my physician told me my blood pressure, cholesterol and triglycerides were too high. Unless I did something different, I was a good candidate for a stroke or heart attack. This was before my wife and I enrolled in Brenda Cobb's Living Foods Lifestyle 10-Day Program one year ago and began a new life.

Six weeks after I started the Living Foods Lifestyle, I had lost

36 pounds and several inches from my waistline. I now have normal blood pressure, cholesterol and triglycerides. People at work have stopped me in the hallway and begged me to tell them what I was doing to cause such a drastic improvement in my appearance and energy. I was thinner, but my doctor told me she noticed that I had fewer lines on my face and I looked younger. Before long, my hair changed color, from white to salt and pepper. My eyes have returned to their original blue, and my vision has improved. I now have a weaker prescription. My chiropractor told me that I adjust easier since I became a Living Foodist.

What was more unexpected was meeting all the wonderful Living/Raw Foodists around the world. I highly recommend the Living Foods Lifestyle to everyone ready to take their life and health to new heights. The Living Foods Lifestyle is the most powerful thing I have ever done!

Nutrient Absorption

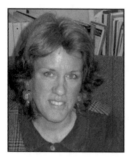

SHERRY WHEAT Atlanta, Georgia
I began taking the 10-day Living Foods class in June 2000. I took the classes over a period of time, and by October I'd completed the majority of the classes.

When I came to the class I was exhausted. Events of the previous two years – getting married and developing a new business – had taken their toll. I wasn't one to experience exhaustion for long periods of time. I didn't feel well and I knew I had to change something about how I ran my life.

Sometimes I would sit quietly in my office at the end of the day and tap into my body. I was aware that my belly was feeling toxic, bloated and congested. A friend who knew I was complaining of this condition told me about Brenda, her story and the Living Foods Lifestyle. I came to a lecture, ate the foods and decided to enroll. Not knowing if the "diet" would have an impact, I was willing to start somewhere.

I was too exhausted to take all the classes at once, so I paced myself, making gradual changes in my food preparation at home. I didn't find it easy. As a victim of habit, some of the easiest things, such as soaking nuts overnight, were highly challenging for me! I started to prepare and eat the easier recipes such as hummus, curried lentil salad and marinated greens. I couldn't bring myself to start making Rejuvelac until October.

As I was eating these specially prepared foods I was more careful about eating raw salads. I began the process of regular colonics and enemas. I used wheatgrass implants, both anally and vaginally. I started to feel better. I noticed that I wasn't quite as exhausted. My body wasn't itching as much as usual. I tested myself and my body. If I went off the diet, I would start to itch more. My bowels became much more regular and frequent, although it took a while for that to happen – probably two to three months. I didn't feel as congested and toxic. I felt "cleaner."

In January I saw Warren Cargal, a friend and a psychotherapist who works in numerous modalities. He suggested I take a saliva and urine test to see what kind of additional support I might need in my recovery process. I took his tests and came in a week later for his analysis. Much to my surprise, and I think to his, my absorbency rating was the highest of any he had ever seen, a benchmark others should be striving for. He made some recommendations and I went on my way. That meant my colon was functioning properly and contributing to the nurturing of my body, that I was absorbing more from my food and that I could rebuild my reserves and energy.

Since that test, I find that I go on and off the diet. I'm actually not ashamed of this! It's just the way it is. Changing food preparation after 50 years is not an easy thing for me. Perhaps if I'd had an immediate, life-threatening condition I'd feel differently. I notice that when I'm off, my colon becomes more sluggish, I itch a little bit more and I'm a little more tired. I'm back on the diet now and incorporate it about 50 percent of the time. I'm more selective when I'm out at friends' homes or at restaurants. My colon responds right away to the change when I go back on raw and Living Foods.

I'm learning how to pace myself in preparing the foods, and how to make the right size batches. (Initially I made batches that were too large and wasted food.) I'm fortunate that my husband likes the food and loves eating what I prepare. I'm thrilled that I have new tools for taking better care of myself and slowing the aging process. I have more energy to continue to build a new business and nurture a new marriage.

My goal now, after my involvement for a year, is to continue to learn and expand my repertoire of recipes, and watch for additional physical, emotional and spiritual changes.

Sherry's acupuncturist felt compelled to make the following statement regarding the urine/saliva test on which her marks were so high.

"Sherry Wheat was seen in our office for acupuncture treatment. As part of the treatment we provide a urine/saliva analysis as an objective analysis of an individual's nutritional and biochemical status in several key areas.

A part of that urine test system is the gut absorption/malabsorption test. This test allows us to screen for the presence of harmful anaerobic bacteria and bowel dysbiosis, a toxic condition caused by a decline in the population of beneficial digestive bacteria. This can lead to malabsorption, digestive disturbances, allergies and inflammatory symptoms.

Sherry had excellent gut absorption test results. This was a surprise for us in the clinic as gut malabsorption is more the typical client profile we see. When we inquired about what she was eating, she informed us that she had been doing the Living Foods program for a number of months. This program appears to be an integral part in helping an individual move to health and vitality."

Warren Cargal, Dipl. Ac., L.Ac., M.A.

ALLERGIES / OSTEOARTHRITIS

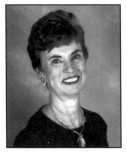

SUSAN TILGHMAN Dunwoody, Georgia
I came to the Living Foods Lifestyle training for several reasons: to lose weight, to get off many of the medications I was taking, and to alleviate symptoms of osteoarthritis in my knees. Guess what – all of this has happened and I'm not even eating 100 percent raw.

My doctor took me off Zocor when I told her about my new way of eating. She literally jumped for joy when she heard I was giving up meat and dairy. I've lost two pants sizes since my course in November 2000 and my knees no longer hurt. My doctor also told me to stop taking the daily prescription antihistamine for allergies. She said I wouldn't be bothered by allergies anymore. She was right.

ARTHRITIS / ALLERGIES / INTUITION

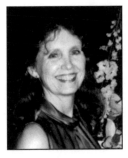

MARY HELEN KING Norcross, Georgia
I took the Living Foods course in October 2000, and continue to eat about 90 percent raw. I've lost weight, have much more energy and require a couple of hours less sleep each night.

In addition, the arthritis in my fingers is showing improvement, an ongoing, nagging cough that has been with me for several years now has gone away and I had almost no allergy symptoms this spring.

Those are just the physical improvements. I have a private energy healing practice and have been quite sensitive to the energy of others for some years now. Since I became a Living Foodist, I find that my intuitions and my ability to sense energy are heightened. I feel an even stronger connection than ever to the "All That Is."Also, several of my friends have noticed my improvements and have asked what I'm doing and have even asked for recipes. I'm grateful to Brenda for this opportunity to learn and grow and improve my life. Thank you again.

EYESIGHT

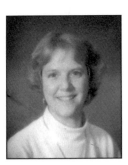

BARBARA ROBERTS Ellijay, Georgia
I took the class in November 2000 and since then I have noticed that my eyes are no longer sensitive to bright sunshine like they used to be. I have temporarily taken a job as a rural postal carrier in Cumming, Georgia, and have to wear reading glasses to see the addresses on the mail. I was worried about how I was going to wear them plus my sunglasses. I tried it and it didn't work well at all with the two of them at the same time.

Then I realized I don't need the sunglasses anymore. This is coming from someone who was so sensitive that I kept a spare pair of sunglasses in my wallet (the flat kind the eye doctor gives you when he dilates your eyes) just in case I lost or broke mine. This is a wonderful, freeing thing because my eyes actually would tear and water in bright sunshine – I couldn't even keep them open, which made driving a bit challenging.

I have noticed that a spot on my face by my nose that was gradually getting larger – to the point that I was considering going to a dermatologist to have it checked out – is definitely shrinking now and getting much lighter since being on Living Foods. I am relieved. I have been blessed to have wonderful health, except for a few minor things, so I feel grateful. I notice since taking the class that I only require six hours of sleep each night. I have to be up at 5:00 or 5:30 a.m. to get to the Post Office and I don't go to bed until 11:00 or 11:30 p.m. When I wake up (usually before the alarm goes off), I am refreshed and well rested, not grumpy and tired as I was before. I love having two extra hours in my day to do the things I want to do. That alone would be worth the price of the class! Keep up the good work educating people!

MENTAL CLARITY

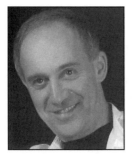

DAVID MOORLAG Roswell, Georgia
I excitedly write to inform you of an apparent increase in my mental clarity and – dare I say – an increase in intelligence. Around the seventh day of my commitment to a totally raw and organic food program I began to notice a calm loving nature was crowding out my usual Capricorn, goal-directed, ambitious personality.

I now feel, after two weeks, decidedly smarter, more intuitive, less scattered and more grounded. If I may humbly submit, I also have a new-felt form of divine guidance and presence. Thank you for teaching so well the spiritual connection between our bodies and our food. I enrolled in your Living Foods class looking for peak performance in my athletic endeavors. I got what I came for and a lot more.

DIABETES / OBESITY

LEO OXLEY College Park, Georgia
I enrolled in the Living Foods Lifestyle Program March 8, 2001. I had three major health concerns: marked obesity, insulin dependent diabetes

(for six years) and marked hypertension. On the second day of the program, my blood sugars dropped to normal levels and continued to be normal, thereby necessitating no insulin or pills to maintain normal blood sugars. After being on the program just a little more than one month – from March 8 to April 17 – I have lost 31 pounds and still have no need for insulin. I haven't seen any influence on my blood pressure to date.

CANCER / JOINT PAIN / LYMPHEDEMA

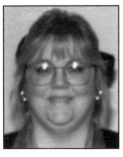

CONNIE COPELAND Norcross, Georgia
I've been trying to find an analogy or something to compare to demonstrate the power and the value of Brenda Cobb and the work she does at the Living Foods Institute.

There's nothing great enough, big enough, grand enough to compare, so I'll simply tell you how completing the program has affected my life:

- My joint pain is gone.
- My teeth feel as if I just had them cleaned at the dentist's office.
- I no longer have body odor. By 5:00 p.m. on a regular workday, I needed to wash and reapply deodorant. Not anymore!
- I sleep like a baby. I turn off the light, go right to sleep and sleep soundly until the alarm goes off. The real joy is no longer waking up during the night and having to go to the bathroom – something I've done for years.
- For years I was plagued with urinary leakage during the day. It has stopped completely.
- My face is clearer and I've been told that it glows.
- My usual food cravings have disappeared.
- I am keenly aware of the mental clarity I now possess. Before, I seemed to give new meaning to the term "brain fog."
- My blood pressure has been steadily dropping.
- The daily swelling in my ankles is gone.
- I'd suffered off and on with depression. It has greatly improved, and I'm looking forward to it going away completely after being on the Living Foods Lifestyle for a while.

- My eyesight has improved. I was sitting at the computer having trouble seeing with the glasses that normally gave me clear vision. When I removed them, I could see the computer screen much better.
- I've lost weight. I don't own a scale because the numbers lost their importance years ago. The way my body feels is what is important. Judging from the way my clothes are fitting, I would estimate from 10 to 15 pounds, possibly more during the 10-day class.
- I had a profound realization as a result of an emotional break-through that has forever changed my life. It has freed me from years of fear and anxiety and has allowed my spirit to soar.
- After having 21 lymph nodes removed during breast surgery, I experienced lymphedema – a swelling from my underarm down to my fingers – for eight months. Nothing relieved the swelling or the extreme pain. After 10 days on Living Foods, my arm was normal, just as before my surgery. All swelling disappeared. The pain in my arm kept me focused on the cancer. When the pain left, I focused on healing and good health.

I came to the Living Foods Institute because of breast cancer. I know, because of the Living Foods Lifestyle, that I will live a long and healthy life. I came for one reason, but have been blessed many times over by the immeasurable joy that has come into my life.

CHRONIC ASTHMA

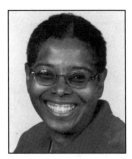

MEREDITH WHITEMAN Snellville, Georgia
I was referred to this program by a good friend who knows I suffer from chronic asthma. I learned that I could heal my problem through the Living Foods Lifestyle. I noticed a change in my chest from day one. By day three most of the wheezing had subsided and I wasn't waking up at night to puff on inhalers. Today, after only 10 days on the program, 90 percent of my coughing is gone. I can take a deep breath without wheezing, and I'm only using my short-acting inhaler twice a day – a major improvement! I'm also walking greater distances without becoming short of breath. My

chest feels strong and the coughing is almost gone.

The quality of my life is improving daily. I'm thrilled with these results in such a short space of time. Other benefits include a lower blood pressure and improvements in the texture of my skin and hair. If I can see this sort of change in 10 days, imagine what can happen over a lifetime. This is definitely the Lifestyle for me. I have finally come home. Thank you, Brenda.

CHOLESTEROL

DEBORAH NEELY Roswell, Georgia

I came to the Living Foods Institute to learn how to prepare raw and Living Foods. They taught me that and so much more! I feel as if a whole new world has opened up for me.

This whole Lifestyle really honors the holistic paradigm I value. Taking seeds through the processes of soaking, planting and/or sprouting to obtain nourishment makes me feel connected to the life force of the planet. Living Foods is the missing piece of my dietary puzzle.

All the staff has been supportive and caring. It's also comforting to know that the support system will be available to me in the future as I explore this new adventure. I definitely plan to volunteer at the Institute.

I've received some bonuses from this program as well – meeting new friends, losing weight and something I didn't expect, lowering my cholesterol 32 points in only 10 days. I want to express my gratitude to the Divine Power, which led me to Living Foods, and a special thank you to Brenda Cobb and the Living Foods Institute.

WEIGHT LOSS / FLEXIBILITY / ENERGY

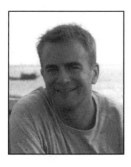

JASON EWING, Atlanta, Georgia
I can't thank you enough for this experience. It really has been amazing. Before I started I thought this would be interesting, but I didn't really expect to change that much. I thought, "Hey, I do Bikram Yoga almost every day. I'm pretty healthy already. I eat right (so I thought), and I try to keep my attitude as positive as possi-

ble for our Yoga students."

Then the first two days hit and I felt terrible. It really made me step back and examine some things. I never realized how much food could affect the body. It explains why my back would break out, the skin chafing/rashes, even acne on my face. I would always say to myself, "I'm 30 years old, and I'm still breaking out?"

You've also shattered the whole protein myth. I was eating way too much protein and my yoga was hurting because of it. I have felt "heavy" since last December, not because of actual weight but because of low energy and "sinking" thoughts. So much of that has lifted now.

My creative energy has returned and I have plans to do things in my apartment and the yoga studio. I've always been a list person and now I know I'll complete them more and more. I also want to clean everything out – my closet, the storage closet at the studio and these boxes I haven't touched since I moved in more than a year ago. They're full of old scraps, mementos and pictures. It hit me the other day that it's time to let go of so much of that, the "things."

During just 10 days I lost 10 pounds and my yoga students noticed. I have increased flexibility and I have had amazing yoga classes. I have a greater sense of joy overall. Music sounds better. Energy! Energy! Energy! I read a quote from Maya Angelou a couple weeks ago that has kept coming up for me during this time, "When you know better, you ought to do better." So now I know!

NUTRITIONAL EDUCATION / IMPROVED ENERGY

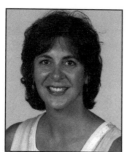

SUSAN HITCHNER Marietta, Georgia
After 13 years of trying to pass on "good eating habits" to my children, I finally know what good eating habits are. It was always difficult for me to find conviction when urging my kids to finish their chicken or their pasta. I would turn away and think to myself, "They don't need chicken. They don't need pasta." And I would give up. The nutritional education I gained through the Living Foods program is priceless. As I go on my "human" way, if I slip off the program, I know the consequences will manifest themselves, just as the benefits have.

As for the spiritual benefits, for once I feel unconditional faith that I can make a change of this magnitude in my life. Sitting in class, I felt doubt lift from my shoulders and fly through the skylight. I learned so much about the potential of human interaction amidst this wonderful, spiritual group of people here – members and employees alike. Along my journey toward enlightenment, I had begun to wonder why I was not attracting like people to myself. I now realize that I have to go where they are, and they're here! In the 10 days I have lost weight; have much improved energy; a greater appreciation for the human spirit; and physical exercise has become more enjoyable. This has been the most positively transforming experience of my life.

SPIRITUAL HEALING / BLOOD PRESSURE / CHOLESTEROL

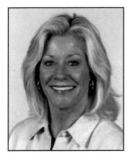

JOY KINCAID Dallas, Texas
I came to this course as a result of finding a lump in my breast (which turned out to be nothing), but I see it as a blessing, because it got me here. I've been health conscious most of my life, but had strayed from my path and wanted to get back on track. I'm amazed at the gifts and blessings I've received from this experience. It has been a life-changing event for me. This course has helped me realize exactly what I want from my life, and that it is totally attainable.

In addition to being a wonderful learning experience with regard to diet and nutrition, this class has been an incredibly spiritual experience. I've gained such clarity with regard to my purpose for being, and I've had the wonderful opportunity to witness amazing breakthroughs mentally, physically, spiritually and emotionally in myself and in those around me.

I can honestly say this is the most amazing experience I've ever had in an environment designed to facilitate personal improvement. In just 10 days I lost 2 percent of my body fat, and my cholesterol dropped 31 points. My pulse rate dropped 20 beats, and my blood pressure dropped as well. This course was an incredible gift, and I would highly recommend it to anyone and everyone! I came to the Living Foods Institute to learn how to nourish my body, and I learned that, but more, I learned how to nourish my mind, my soul and my spirit, those around me and ultimately, the planet. I came to the Living Foods Institute to learn how to eat. I learned that, but more important, I learned how to live!

HEADACHES / RHEUMATOID ARTHRITIS / SUGAR CRAVING

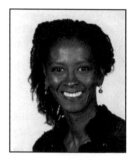

B.K. Atlanta, Georgia

I've always considered myself to be in good health. Checkups were always good, etc. I've also always known that we are beings of a higher nature than we allow ourselves to be, but have strayed from that knowledge.

About 14 months ago I developed a headache in the lower right side of my head that was present in varying degrees 24 hours a day. I am not a "headache person." At the same time, starting several years ago, I was having increasing pain in my lower right back radiating up and down the whole right side. I experienced some relief through chiropractic sessions, but increasingly found myself waking up in the mornings and feeling as though a large ball had dropped to the bottom of my right lower back and having to roll myself out of bed. The headache was also worse upon waking. I had been diagnosed with rheumatoid arthritis and a deteriorating right hip, and told I would just have to learn to live with the pain. MRIs and blood tests for the headache found nothing, but there was a small tumor on my right ovary. I was also having severe hot flashes and night sweats, waking up every two hours every night.

I was "guided" to this Center and the spirituality residing here. After just 10 days, my headache is gone. I no longer have acute pain in my back, nor do I have to roll out of bed. I'm getting back in touch and becoming reconnected to my intuitive being and am experiencing a calm and inner peace. I also no longer crave the refined sugar and other harmful substances that I've loved for more than 30 years. Oh, and no more hot flashes and night sweats! I've been about 75 percent raw and Living for about three months and I am getting better and better in too many ways to list. I feel more in touch with life and (I'm told by friends and family) I'm truly happier, healthier and more loving.

BELL'S PALSY

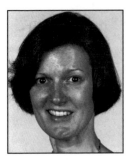

CRISSY BRAND Alpharetta, Georgia
I was just 12 years old when it happened ... It was the day after Christmas and my cousin and I were trying on our new Bonne Belle Lip Smacker lip gloss in her bedroom. That's when it happened! I wasn't able to rub my lips together after applying the gloss. My cousin looked at me and started screaming. My face was paralyzed on the left side and it happened in an instant. My mother rushed me to the small hospital in Harrisonburg, Virginia. The doctors didn't know why half my face had suddenly become paralyzed. I was scared, and my mother was scared for me.

It wasn't until we got back to Atlanta after the holidays and went to a neurologist that I found out what had happened to my face was called Bell's Palsy – a paralysis of the face. For the next several months I had to tape my left eye shut at night because I couldn't close it and keep it closed voluntarily. I used liquid tears all day long because my left eye couldn't blink on its own. I talked, ate, smiled and laughed only out of the right side of my mouth. I looked like Popeye the Sailorman. Kids in school were very cruel and the paralysis was humiliating. Over the next months, my face gradually improved until it leveled out to a partial paralysis that plagued me for the next 22 years.

I met Brenda Cobb in February 2001 after my mother was diagnosed with breast cancer. I went to hear her story about curing herself of breast and cervical cancer by changing her diet and lifestyle to the Living Foods Lifestyle. While I was listening to her story, I thought maybe she could help me with the severe food allergies and asthma I'd developed over the past few years. I decided to take the 10-Day Program at the Living Foods Institute to see if this Lifestyle would help me. On day two of the class, I was able to eat foods I'd been allergic to for years – with no allergic reaction. On day six of the class, I decided I wanted to adopt the Living Foods Lifestyle as my own. That was only a few short months ago, and I've never felt better – or younger – in my life.

The next wonderful thing that happened is that my daughter Nicole started noticing the changes in my life. She became very interested in the Living Foods Lifestyle and asked me if she could also take the 10-day class at the Living Foods Institute. The miracle in her question is that she is only 13 years old. I knew I could never force this Lifestyle on her because she is a teenager. She did take the 10-day class and it has changed her life and her thinking. She has been given the beautiful gift of a healthy, happy life. When she has children, they will never know an unhealthy day in their lives.

A good friend came to visit me recently. She kept looking at me and commenting that I looked different. She said my skin had changed and looked beautiful, but that wasn't what was different. After some time, she told me the difference was that the paralysis from my Bell's Palsy was better. I couldn't believe her words and went to the bathroom mirror to smile and see for myself. My left eye used to close almost completely when I smiled, chewed, laughed or cried. My eye is no longer closing. A few days later, I was on the phone with another friend and realized I could whistle – something I haven't been able to do for 22 years. I started crying tears of joy. I can now hold water in my mouth without it spilling out the left side, and I can hold air in my mouth. For me, this is a miracle – a dream come true! In addition to my Bell's Palsy improving, my allergies and asthma have completely gone away. I also sleep two to three hours less every night with more energy than I've ever had. What other wonderful things are going to happen in my life because I've adopted the Living Foods Lifestyle?

I have Brenda Cobb to thank for making it her life's work to share this Lifestyle with other people. Thank you Brenda, Rich, Joanne, Ann and Reed! You've all been a part of changing my life. I can hardly wait to see what other wonderful things are in store for me!

WEIGHT / BODY FAT

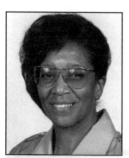

DELORIS HAYNES Atlanta Georgia

I came because I love clean living. I want to look right, live right and eat right. I don't want to allow a medical doctor to tell me what to do or control my body and health.

I came from a large family of 11 children. I'm 56, the second-oldest child still living in my family. A brother died at age 42 of a massive heart attack. Four months later a sister died of colon cancer. A year later my 49-year-old sister died of a heart attack. A year later, my 52-year-old sister died from lung problems, diabetes and goiter. The doctor said we have hereditary heart disease.

During these 10 days I made up my mind that I'm going to have perfect health and any problem I may have had will be healed. All my siblings are under doctor's care, and they're always trying to get me to go see the doctor for a growth behind my ear. I refused. I'm now eating Living Foods and I believe I will be completely healed. I thought I was coming to learn how to prepare foods only, but this has been the most spirit-filled 10-day class I have been in. I've been motivated beyond measure. I missed Sunday school while in class and was feeling bad about it. But I came to class and we had such a spirit-filled time I felt great when I left. I didn't miss a thing, and the staff – I could never say enough about them. They're great. In the 10 days, I lost weight, and my body fat went down. I'm feeling great and others are telling me I look so much better. I feel better about myself. I had dark circles around my eyes; they are gone. Most of all, I'm thankful for the knowledge I have about Living Foods. I know what to put into my body in order to be healthy.

MIXED TUMOR ADENOMA

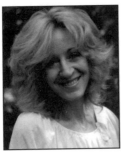

SUSAN AHL PIPER Stone Mountain, Georgia Six years ago, I was found to have mixed tumor adenoma in my right parotid (major salivary gland). A superficial parotidectomy was performed, removing the diseased tissue. Eight months ago, I felt a small tumor in the hinge of my right mandible. A biopsy found this tumor was a recurrence of the earlier tumor. After an MRI, my oncologist gave me two options: radiation or a total parotidectomy. He said the total parotidectomy had some risk, as four branches of the facial nerve grow through that organ.

When I began telling friends what was going on with me, one friend, Glenn (whose girlfriend was a former student of the Living Foods Institute), suggested I consider eating raw foods. I immediately went to the introductory class and meal the following weekend. I told my story, and Brenda suggested I not eat nuts, sweet fruits or concentrated foods on my healing regimen, a restriction she suggested for cancer patients. I began reading about raw foods and Ann Wigmore, and talking to people who cured themselves of cancer with raw foods.

Five months ago I went on 100 percent raw and organic food, with the occasional addition of spelt bread to my diet. I also bought a Jupiter filter around the second month and within two weeks I was drinking 9.0 alkaline water supplemented with 900 milligrams per day of Transfer Factor and 1000 milligrams per day of Beta Glucan. My diet has consisted daily of 2 ounces of fresh, squeezed wheatgrass juice prior to breakfast, fresh avocados and apples for breakfast, and salad with fresh vegetables, sprouts, avocados and sunflower seeds for lunch/dinner with homemade dressing consisting of flaxseed oil, lemon juice, garlic, sea salt and stevia, with fresh fruit throughout the day – and lots of water. I eat no GMO foods (no tomatoes, carrots, potatoes or other root vegetables, and no soy products). I have professional colonics every two weeks.

- One month into my regimen, my skin was glowing from the cleanse.
- Three months into my regimen, my digestive system began to heal after about 15 years of disease.
- Four months into my regimen, all of my premenopausal symptoms disappeared (hot flashes and sweats) and severe menstrual cramps, which I'd had since age 12, disappeared.
- Five months into my regimen, my parotid tumor disappeared. You may be interested in knowing that at the date of this writing, the oncologist who diagnosed my tumor and wanted to operate has confirmed the healing and released me from his care.

Again, I thank you, Brenda, for your guidance and for being such an inspiration.

BREAST CANCER

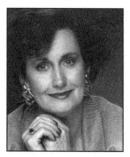

SHIRLEY HIGHTOWER Marietta, Georgia
I was diagnosed with breast cancer in May 2000. I immediately began researching alternative treatments and found out about Ann Wigmore and the Living Foods Lifestyle. This natural healing approach just made good sense to me. I found out that Brenda Cobb had a Living Foods program in Atlanta and I immediately called and enrolled for her 10-Day Detoxification and Rebuilding Program. In just the first 10 Days I began to feel much better. I found the support I needed at the Institute and I lost about 7 pounds.

When first diagnosed my tumor was a 2.1. After doing the Living Foods Lifestyle for about 30 days I had a lumpectomy in June 2000. When the doctor removed the lump it was only a 1.4. So, in that small amount of time my tumor shrank. Before surgery I was told I would have to at least have radiation and possibly chemotherapy, but when I returned to the oncologist I found that I wouldn't need any chemotherapy or radiation. I believe that is a direct result of the Living Foods Lifestyle.

Besides the wonderful results with cancer I have also experienced better sleep, much higher energy, my hair became shinier with thicker texture, my skin became beautiful, glowing and young looking, and my attitude became very positive.

The Lord has truly blessed me. I am so glad that I found the Living Foods Institute and I thank them and Brenda Cobb for the positive, encouraging support.

TYPICAL CLASS RESULTS

At the end of each 10-day Program, we ask our students to give us a testimonial and a list of the improvements they have seen. Every class notes incredible improvements. These results from a recent class are representative of what we hear from students again and again:

Weight Loss	Increased Flexibility	More Energy
Sense of Joy	Better and Deeper Sleep	Improved Lungs
Lessened Allergies	Sharpened Senses	More Patient
Lower Blood Pressure	Emotionally Stable	Restored Faith
More Peaceful	Mystical Experience	Lower Body Fat
Better Attitude	Lower Cholesterol	More Intuitive
More Positive	Hot Flashes Ceased	No Migraines
Improved Appearance	Physiological Improvement	Feel Lighter
Color Returned to Face	No Craving for Sweets	Eating Less
More Hopeful	More Appreciative	Softer Skin
Cellulite Vanishing	Emotional Baggage Released	Calmness
Became Reconnected	Acute Back Pain Gone	Look Younger
Enhanced Meditation	Pulse Rate Dropped	Clearer Skin
Improved Digestion	Spiritual Awareness	More Productive

During the 10-Day Training each month we measure cholesterol, blood pressure and weight on the first day of training and again on the ninth day. The results are dramatic, as you will see. The following statistics are actual test results for our students. For the purpose of this chart, we are using the initials of the students tested.

Student Initials	Cholesterol Day 1	Cholesterol Day 9	Weight Day 1	Weight Day 9	Blood Pressure Day 1	Blood Pressure Day 9
MG	213	158				
CP	216	156				
MG					153/100	121/76
AC	242	185	197	185		
RS			258	241		
PM			241	230		
DH	205	154				
SM	226	170				
LD	251	190				
BS	239	155	221.5	210		
RS					131/119	120/107
JM					124/92	95/77
VM	232	160				
CH	203.6	192				
LC	239.4	225.6				
JW	270	152				
TK			210.2	199.6		
JJ	199	157				
SB			163	152		
DB			196	177.8		
MP			174.8	162.2		
TJ	217	177				
RJ					143/92	138/86
NR			164.2	153.2		

Student Initials	Cholesterol Day 1	Cholesterol Day 9	Weight Day 1	Weight Day 9	Blood Pressure Day 1	Blood Pressure Day 9
OW					145/99	124/88
RC					134/83	112/73
DR	233	156				
PB					157/101	118/74
AT					123/83	106/70
JJ	222	164				
SL			223.4	211		
TD	198	150				
MG					193/114	156/91
JG					144/108	113/71
LG	211	150	248.4	236	144/108	134/84
KH					151/106	127/86
BS	181	150			151/106	92/68
BM	216	177	215	205		
LE	215	188				
PL	249	206				
NB	275	218				
DB	205	150				

CHAPTER TWO

MY STORY

Then God said, "I give you every seed bearing plant on the face of the whole earth and every tree that has fruit with seed in it. They will be yours for food. And to all the beasts of the earth and all the birds of the air and all the creatures that move on the ground – everything that has the breath of life in it – I give every green plant for food." – Genesis 1:29

WITHOUT MY HEALTH, WHAT DID I HAVE?

It was a cloudy day in February 1999, and warmer than usual. I had trouble finding a parking space at the doctor's office and had to drive around until someone finally left. I've never cared for doctors' offices. Everyone looks unhappy, the sights are depressing and I can't stand the smell. It seemed as if I waited forever for the nurse to call my name. She escorted me to the scale. I almost fell off it when I weighed in at 192 pounds. I felt fat. I looked fat. I was fat. The scale confirmed it; I was out of control. Having no scale in my home had helped me avoid the horrible truth. I was "Miss Piggy." Oink, oink.

I've never been comfortable going to the doctor. Thoughts of doctors' offices and hospitals have always brought up unpleasant memories and fear. When I was a baby I received vaccinations in both my thighs. I had a reaction to the medication and the sites of the shots festered into boils. Even though I was a baby, I can remember the pain of having those boils lanced. I screamed bloody murder, and I still have scars to remind me of that pain.

I also remember terrible earaches when I was little and getting more shots. I remember allergies so bad I couldn't play outside during certain times of the year without constantly sneezing and coughing. I remember what seemed like hundreds of allergy tests throughout the years, along with more shots and more doctor visits.

I also remember the nurses who gave me those shots. One in particular was cold, hateful and made fun of me when I told her I thought I was going to faint. I was only nine at the time, but that image remains.

I remember the first time I saw my father in intensive care. At 42 he'd had his first heart attack and tubes were coming out of him everywhere. Seeing someone I loved so much in this frightening state made me feel sick to my stomach. Again, I thought I was going to faint, so I told a nurse. Instead of empathy or even sympathy, I was yelled at and chastised for being weak.

My relationships with medical professionals have not been great. For me to visit a doctor, something has to be wrong. Something was very wrong that day in February. I remember exactly what the doctor said, with a distressed look and a note of alarm in his voice, "You better be glad you came in here when you did. This visit could have just saved your life."

He was right! It did save my life, but not because I took his recommendation to have surgery – because it led me to the Living Foods Lifestyle! I believe everything happens for a reason, and no matter how bad a situation may appear, there is good in it if we look for it. Much good has come from my health challenges; I have grown and healed in many ways. I adopted the Living Foods Lifestyle to get rid of breast and cervical tumors, but I got much more – I got a brand new life!

Without health, we can't truly enjoy life. The state of our health makes the difference in whether we get the most out of life or just barely make it through. Are you running, jumping and skipping through life, or are you dragging those legs behind you, feeling like you have "one foot in the grave"? Almost everyone I know wants to feel good so they can enjoy life and be active. I've discovered joy through my own search for perfect health, and I truly enjoy every moment of every day because I feel so good.

A SOUTHERN ADDICTION

I've lived in the South all my life. I was born to a family that loved food and knew how to fix it. I enjoyed good ol' Southern dishes such as fried chicken, macaroni and cheese, collard greens, rice and gravy, corn bread and pecan pie. My mother made the best cakes in the world – German chocolate, coconut and chocolate layer. Every family gathering centered on food, and with lots of good cooks in the family, holidays were a smorgasbord of goodies. We had sweet potato, lemon meringue and blackberry pies, mashed potatoes and gravy, country-fried steak, pot roast, baked ham and potato salad. Sometimes we had all these foods and more at one meal, especially at Christmas and Thanksgiving. One of my aunts made the best macaroni and cheese in the world, and I always looked forward to family gatherings so I could eat my fill. For breakfast we ate bacon, sausage, ham, grits, eggs and biscuits. In summer we made ice cream and barbecued chicken. Food was the focus of our lives – we'd talk about what we were going to have for dinner while we were still eating lunch.

STARVING TO DEATH FOR BEAUTY

Needless to say, with all the interest in food, I was an overweight child. This caused me much embarrassment. Not until junior high school, when I became interested in boys, did I decide to do something about my weight. That's when I began a lifetime of dieting. As a teenager I starved myself on the grapefruit diet, skipping meals in an effort to take the weight off. I'd lose it, then I'd gain it back plus some. I was obsessed with food, or the lack of it, and most every waking hour I was thinking about what I could or couldn't eat. I jumped on the scales every day or so, panicking when I gained an ounce and crying when I hadn't lost any. During all that time, I never thought about the nutritional value of food. All I thought about was the calories, and how few I could get by on. I survived – barely – on 500 or fewer calories a day for weeks at a time.

Every moment I was starving myself to death, I was also thinking about food. When I couldn't take dieting anymore I would binge on every food I could stuff in my mouth. It's a good thing I didn't like to throw up, or surely I would have become bulimic. Instead, I dieted and binged for years, losing and gaining the same weight over and over.

At 16 I entered my first beauty pageant and life became an endless battle to keep the weight off. I exercised. I starved. I weighed myself every day. I pretended I was happy and carefree, but inside I was miserable because I was a slave to food. I gained a lot through competing in pageants, from poise and confidence to scholarship money, but the constant battle to stay thin almost drove me crazy.

Most of my life I ate the Standard American Diet (SAD). I now know why they call it the SAD diet. It brings misery and disease to people and to the animals that are slaughtered for their flesh. I've eaten my share of cows, chicken, pigs, fish, seafood and even the occasional squirrel or deer, but I'm not proud of it. I'm sorry I ever ate an animal, and I'm glad I don't eat them anymore. Animals are our friends. I don't eat anything with a face, and I never will again.

GROUNDS FOR DIVORCE

In my late 20s, after divorcing my first husband, a pharmacist, I became more interested in health and nutrition. I began to search for the perfect diet. Still, my emphasis was on losing weight, not gaining health. I tried the Atkins Diet, the Hilton Head Diet, the Grapefruit Diet, the Stars Diet, Body Ecology, Eat Right For Your Blood Type, Macrobiotics, Vegetarianism and Veganism – and those are just the ones I remember. Despite all the diets, I still struggled with my weight. After the birth of my son Rich, my weight really became a problem. Every year I would add – and keep – two or three pounds. I'd balloon up to 150 or 160 pounds, crash diet down to 120 or 130 pounds, and then start all over again. Weight was the focus of my life. Add all the weight together, and I've gained and lost at least one entire person.

I realize now that my eating was never in control, and it got more out of control at certain periods of my life. I got married when I was 19. My mother tried to tell me I was too young to get married, but I wouldn't listen. I weighed 112 pounds and had a good figure.

My ex-husband said that if I got fat, it was grounds for divorce. I worried about my weight throughout my marriage. I didn't eat in front of my husband because he criticized me and commented on every bite I took. I made excuses not to sit at the table. I told him I wasn't hungry, I'd already eaten or I was dieting. He said, "That's good. You know what'll happen if you get fat. I'd hate to divorce you."

Watching my figure didn't stop me from getting a divorce when Rich was only three months old. I only gained about 15 pounds while I was pregnant, and I'd lost all that weight and had my figure back. But getting a divorce after almost nine years of marriage was stressful, so I ate. I also needed a job to support Rich and myself. I began working in a trendy, late-night restaurant so I could care for him during the day. I sampled all the tempting food and drinks the restaurant had to offer. I ate filet mignon, escargot, duck, chocolate mousse, cherry cheesecake and every other delicious dish from that temperamental French chef.

Then I began having an occasional cocktail, some new, exciting concoction the bartender had just created. One drink led to two, and then to three. Then I was having a drink every day after work. I ate late and I ate lots. The food at the restaurant was wonderful and I tried each dish again and again! Being around all the great food and tasty drinks was just the thing to fuel my addiction. Working in that restaurant helped me pay the bills, and it helped me to get even more out of control and addicted to food.

RIDING THE DEPRESSION CIRCUIT

As Rich got older I changed careers, becoming an interior decorator. I worked long hours and attended endless social functions, where I ate and I drank. My life was a series of appointments, parties, business meetings, drinks and pigs in a blanket. I was determined to "make it" in life and I did it through work. I wanted to be the best, and I would do anything to succeed. I had to mix and mingle, and I did plenty of it. Everything I did revolved around making money and eating. After a long day's work, food and alcohol were the only comfort I could find. I gained weight. Then I lost it for the second, third or fourth time. Do you see how miserable and out of control I was?

I was also depressed. I did a great job of hiding it; most people who knew me then would probably never have guessed I hurt so much. I even fooled myself into thinking everything was OK. After all, I never took drugs for depression; I turned to food and drink instead.

After 12 years as a decorator I changed careers again. I opened a production company and recording studio, thinking that would make me happy. For a while it seemed to work. I was financially successful, but I still used food and drink to compensate for the long hours and empty feelings I had about my life – and myself. I was successful on the outside, but falling apart on the inside. I pretended everything was wonderful when it wasn't. I fooled myself sometimes, but reality would hit and I'd fall into an even deeper depression. When I was low, I was really low.

A CHANGE FOR THE BETTER

This went on for many years before my life began to turn around. After being divorced for 22 years, I remarried in October 1998. My husband Ken is a wonderful man who is both good to me and good for me. Ken and I had known one another and worked together for a number of years. We were great friends first before we fell in love – I believe that's why our marriage is wonderful.

I guess I had listened to my first husband threaten to divorce me if I got fat so many times that I had to pinch myself to believe it was really true that someone could love me even if I was fat. I came to realize that how fat or thin I am doesn't really matter when someone really loves me, but on my wedding day all I could think of was how wonderful my husband-to-be was for loving me although I weighed 185 pounds at the time.

Even at the wedding I couldn't stop thinking about how fat I was. I'd spent months making my own wedding dress and it was exquisite, but I felt fat in it. I was happy to be married, but still unhappy with how I looked and felt. My energy and self-esteem were low; my weight and depression were high. I felt worse about myself every day. I was unhealthy because of my habits and thoughts, the food I ate and the alcohol I drank. I wanted to blame my poor health on anyone but me, but the truth is I was responsible for my own misery and my poor health.

THE REST OF MY STORY

In February 1999, when I went to the doctor for a checkup, I was experiencing heavy bleeding and just didn't feel good. I was depressed, tired, emotionally drained. I had no energy. In other words, I was a mess.

That day changed my life forever. The first bad news was that I weighed in at 192 pounds. At barely 5 feet, 5 inches tall, I was fat! I knew I was fat, but I didn't know just how fat because I didn't have any scales at home – an indication of the depth of my denial. I didn't want to step on the scales. It would've been too much of a shock! I lived most of my life feeling conscious about my weight, stepping on the scales sometimes two or three times a day. I grew to hate the scales and sold them in a yard sale for $3. I never wanted to see a pair of scales again. I was tired of being a prisoner to pounds.

My weight problem alone was bad enough, but the diagnosis soon got worse. The doctor found a large lump in my left breast and a large clump of tumors on my cervix. He was alarmed and recommended surgery immediately. This alarmed me too. The look on his face and the tone of his voice were enough to push me to tears. He sent me to two other doctors who ran additional tests, and they all agreed I should have immediate surgery. Because of the high incidence of cancer in my family (my mother and some of her sisters had breast, ovarian and/or uterine cancer), I'd been told I was at high risk of developing these diseases. With my diagnosis, all my fears came true.

For two days the doctors ran test after test. I spent hours in the hospital waiting for results. That gave me time to think and watch the people around me. I thought about how much I hated hospitals and how I didn't want to spend any more time in one. I watched person after person going in and out of the testing rooms. They all looked depressed. I knew how they felt, because I was depressed too. The longer I sat in that hospital, the worse I felt. I couldn't wait to get out of that depressing environment. I decided that day to take my power back and not to become a victim of the mainstream medical community.

Over the years I'd seen relatives and friends with cancer have surgery, endure chemotherapy and radiation, and suffer the devastating side effects – hair and energy loss, nausea, fatigue, early menopause and many other terrible side effects. I'd seen cancer return or invade other parts of the body, requiring more surgery and treatment. I didn't feel surgery and drugs were for me. I didn't believe they could heal me. And then the doctor said, "Just sign this consent form and when we operate we'll take whatever body parts we need to.

We won't know what all we'll have to remove until we get in there." That's when I knew I wasn't going down that path.

SOMETHING SO RIGHT

I knew I had to address the root cause – how I got into such bad shape in the first place. I also knew I would need to make major changes in my life if I wanted to be healthy and happy again. That's when I discovered the Living Foods Lifestyle. I walked into a health food store and asked one of the employees, "Do you know of any books about healing cancer in a natural way?" She recommended *How I Conquered Cancer Naturally* by Eydie Mae. I was inspired by this courageous woman's story, and I knew intuitively that this natural way of healing was the way I should go. If it worked for her, it might work for me too.

Have you ever read or heard something that just felt right to you? Even if everyone else thought you were crazy, it didn't matter, because you knew it would work? That was how I felt when I read about the Living Foods Lifestyle. I was careful not to talk about my "disease" to others. Though I knew they might mean well, I was concerned that they would try to talk me out of doing something so drastic as making a lifestyle change rather than having surgery and taking chemo. Instead I listened to my inner voice and accepted what it said. This was my first step toward taking back my power. The doctors were telling me I was crazy for not having surgery and taking drugs, but I stayed centered and focused on what I knew would work for me. They even wanted to bring my husband in and make him talk me into surgery. I told them I would make my own decisions about my health and my body and that no one would talk me into anything!

In May 1999 I went to the Ann Wigmore Foundation in New Mexico to learn more about the Living Foods Lifestyle. I read as many books as I could about the Lifestyle before I went to New Mexico, but nothing could've prepared me for the shock I received when I first tried Energy Soup, Rejuvelac and Vege-Kraut.

These "main foods for healing" were what they expected me to eat? They wanted me to eat way more than I could possibly force down, which was anything more than a tablespoon. They talked to me about bowel movements and the importance of cleaning out my colon. At first I was embarrassed, because no one had ever talked so plainly to me about my bodily functions. After a while it became second nature. I had no idea what I was doing the first time I tried to give myself an enema, but I followed the instructions as best I could. It was funny and sad at the same time, but pretty soon I became comfortable with my enema bag. Thank goodness – if I had refused to clean out my colon, I would never have healed.

At first I hated the thought of giving myself enemas or letting someone else give me a colonic. My mind and my body tried to resist, but something within me kept saying, "You have to do this." Despite my aversions, I stuck with it. In two weeks my bleeding had stopped and I had lost 23 pounds. The tumor in my breast began to shrink. I felt lighter, clear-headed, happy and not depressed. My indigestion and acid reflux were gone and I wasn't stopped up with mucous or plagued with allergies.

In just two short weeks I felt like a new woman. You should have seen the look on my husband's face when I arrived back home. He was amazed at how different I looked. The changes were dramatic, and this was just the beginning. Not only was my body healing on the inside, I was changing on the outside too.

Those first two weeks in New Mexico were just the beginning of my healing process. We can't undo in a few days or weeks what it has taken a lifetime to create. I had a lot of work ahead of me, and I have to say it was the biggest challenge of my life. My visit to New Mexico got me started, but when I came home, reality hit. I realized how much I didn't know. I knew I wanted to follow this Lifestyle because I'd seen it bring about great results in a short time. However, I didn't know where to begin. I struggled through the recipes, making every mistake possible. I cried when I poured up my first batch of Rejuvelac, "the water of the Living Foods Lifestyle." It tasted disgusting. I thought I would starve to death before I learned how to make the food. Then I got out my books, read some more and tried to get it right!

During my trial and error approach, and throughout my many disappointments, I kept wishing for someone to show me how to do everything right. I wished for classes I could take – a place I could go for help. But there were no classes or places that I knew of, so I stumbled along. One day, after many failures, I finally figured out how to make Rejuvelac, Energy Soup and Vege-Kraut. After doing dozens of enemas, I realized they had become second nature to me.

A HEALING VISION

One day, when my energy was at an all-time high and I felt clear-headed and focused, I had a vision. There was no place in Atlanta where people could go to learn how to prepare raw and Living Foods and live the Lifestyle. I decided I should open such a place to teach people and help them heal. My life had improved so much because of the Living Foods Lifestyle that I felt I had to share this information with others. And that's how the Living Foods Institute came to be.

I wanted a Living Foods Institute where we could teach people how to live the Lifestyle with ease. I wanted to show them how to put the principles into practice in their full, busy lives and how to keep it simple. I wanted a place where people could learn to prepare healing foods by receiving hands-on instruction in an actual kitchen. I wanted to teach them to release their past and their old habits; to help them make the transition from the Standard American Diet to a new way of thinking about, preparing and combining raw and Living Foods to help the body to heal. I wanted a place where healing was approached from the body, mind and spirit perspective.

What started out as a negative experience, my cancer diagnosis, turned into a positive entity for me and for others. If I hadn't become ill, I would never have opened the Living Foods Institute. What seemed terrible at the time became the most positive thing that has ever happened to me. This proves there is a positive aspect to every situation. No matter how bad it seems at the time, there is always hope. Everything happens for a reason.

DO WHAT'S RIGHT FOR YOU!

When I decided to adopt the Living Foods Lifestyle instead of having surgery or taking drugs, some people, such as my doctors, thought I was crazy. They made no efforts to hide their feelings. But it didn't matter what they thought. I knew what was right for me and I stuck to my decision.

My friends' and relatives' experiences with cancer helped me make my decision and stand by it with conviction. A friend who underwent surgery for breast cancer had a horrible time with subsequent chemotherapy. The side effects were horrendous. She went through early menopause and gained weight. She lost her hair and energy. She was a wreck. A year or so after her treatment, she was still struggling with the side effects of all those poisonous drugs. Seeing what she went through made me even more confident that I would not have surgery or take drugs.

Listen to your inner voice. Make your own decisions about what's right for you. Don't let others' convictions and feelings get in the way of deciding what is best for you. Even those with the best intentions, such as family members and friends, can bombard you with what they think you should do. That can be confusing, especially if what they're saying and what you're thinking are two different things. Always honor your own inner voice. It will never lead you wrong. If it doesn't feel right, don't do it! Stand in your own power. You have all your own answers deep inside you.

YOU GET OUT OF IT WHAT YOU PUT INTO IT

As I mentioned earlier, I didn't tell my family – other than my husband and my son – or my friends that I had cancer before I was completely healed. I knew that if I told them about my decision to try Living Foods instead of surgery they would try to talk me out of it. One friend in particular was skeptical when she found out later what I'd done. A doctor friend of hers believed it wasn't possible for me to heal myself without surgery and drugs, and my friend doubted it herself. She saw how much weight I'd lost – from 192 pounds to 117 pounds – and instead of being happy for me, she said she was worried. Her doctor friend told her that when cancer metastasizes it causes weight loss. She feared that had happened to me. I assured her I was in total and perfect health, but it didn't erase the look of horror on her face.

She called me sometimes, complaining about her weight, low energy and sugar cravings. She'd ask me what I thought she should do. Every time she called I recommended that she take my Living Foods Lifestyle course and put it to work in her life. At that time she resisted the program, but continued to complain about feeling bad and ask me what else she could do. I knew it just wasn't time for her yet, so I continued to send her unconditional love and do spiritual work and prayers for her healing.

She finally signed up for the course, but she seemed resistant to the information and constantly questioned if the program would work. I think she wanted to believe, but her faith wavered. My friend was much like me – we were both addicted to sugar, flour and other bad foods. I think she – as many of us sometimes do – resisted because it meant she would have to change, and change can be scary. But once we realize what we've been doing isn't right or good for us, we know we have to change if we want our health back.

Also, many people let others influence them to the point of confusion. They may believe one thing inside but hear something totally different from friends, relatives or other well-meaning people. This woman's doctor friend was constantly feeding her information that conflicted with what she was learning in class. When I told her she needed enemas and colonics, she disagreed. When I taught her about the dangers of eating meat, she objected and argued that she needed it for protein.

Though my friend seemed somewhat close-minded from the first day of training to the last, she still showed up for class each day. At the graduation party, as other students shared their successes – typically saying how great they felt, how wonderful the training was and how it was the most important thing they'd ever done for them-selves – she still seemed skeptical and unenthusiastic. I understand now that she was doing the best she could at the time, and that it was-n't my responsibility to "fix" her. I wanted to help her because I love her, but I realized I couldn't help her until she was ready to help her-self. So I sent her unconditional love.

After the class was over she called and said she thought she was feeling better and that maybe she would get a Vita-Mix and wheatgrass juicer and try to make more of the foods at home. I was glad she was beginning to see results, and I encouraged her, but still I knew that anything she did had to be her decision and not a result of my persuasion.

I tell you this because there may be someone you want to help, and they may be resistant. Pushing these people won't do any good. Unless a person decides they want to change, no one on earth can change them. We mustn't judge people for their decisions, because each of us is on our own path. We must honor that. We all have our own lessons to learn and challenges to meet. Your responsibility is to yourself and your own healing.

On the other hand, if you decide to do the Living Foods

Lifestyle for yourself and others try to talk you out of it, criticize what you're doing or say you're crazy, remember that you have to do what you think is right for you. Embrace your own power and listen to your inner voice. Do what you want to do, even if everyone around you is trying to convince you otherwise. Your intuition will never lead you wrong. Also, when seeking a program, lifestyle change or diet to follow, look at the person promoting that program. How do they look? Did they get good results? Are they a walking testimony that the program works? If you want to lose weight, you wouldn't ask advice from someone who was overweight, would you? Look for the best example of results and follow it. Don't just believe what everyone says they think will work. Talk to others who have tried the program and see what their results were.

GREAT RESULTS, FAST

In the first six months after adopting the Living Foods Lifestyle, I noticed dramatic results. What began as a quest to get rid of breast and cervical tumors turned out to be a life-changing experience in ways I never expected. As my tumors melted away, my body began to heal from the inside out. It seems everything that was wrong with me fixed itself. Probably things I didn't know were wrong got fixed too. No matter what is going on with you, remember that the Living Foods Lifestyle restores health on every level, both the expected and the unexpected.

I've worked with hundreds of students who've had all types of health problems, and I have seen the remarkable results they experience. They come to class because they have cancer or some other serious disease, and when they begin to heal everything else gets better. They tell me their depression disappeared and their eyesight improved. They talk about how relieved they are that their indigestion and acid reflux are gone, and how their skin has cleared up.

It can happen to anyone who embraces this Lifestyle and really believes it will work. I've seen it happen hundreds of times and it doesn't surprise me at all anymore. There's no secret to it; there's no special club that only a few are privileged to join. Anyone who wants to heal and practices the Living Foods Lifestyle can heal. It all begins in the mind. Belief and faith are powerful healers and can produce miracles.

I believe all disease comes from toxicity and deficiency in the body, the mind and the spirit. Therefore, if we detoxify and rebuild the body, it stands to reason that the body will heal itself. If we detox the mind, the mind will heal. If we detox the spirit, the spirit will heal. Detoxification is an important, necessary part of the Living Foods Lifestyle.

We can name diseases and symptoms anything we want – cancer, heart disease, diabetes, hypoglycemia, lupus, high blood pressure, migraine headaches, Parkinson's Disease, arthritis, sinus, allergies, etc. In truth, these are just fancy names for a toxic body that's deficient in enzymes. We can only heal when we detoxify our body and build it back up with enzymes and other nutrients.

When you are willing to make changes in what you do, you will get changes in your life. Here's a summary of everything that improved with me within the first six months:

- Tumors dissolved.
- Lost 75 pounds.
- Eyesight greatly improved. I no longer need glasses for my distant vision, and my close-up vision is improving, although I do still use my reading glasses.
- Most of my gray hair turned back to its original color.
- Hair became thicker, shinier and grew faster.
- Some wrinkles disappeared completely; others softened.
- Depression vanished.
- Energy level increased 100 percent or more.
- Slept soundly through the night without having to get up to go to the bathroom.
- Hot flashes ceased.
- PMS stopped.
- Bleeding from cervical tumors stopped completely.
- Menstrual flow became light (formerly 7 to 10 days; then 2 to 3 days, then 1 day).
- Age or liver spots on hands and arms disappeared.
- Arthritis went away.
- Skin improved, became clearer, glowing and tanned easily.
- Became increasingly clear-headed and more focused.
- Smell, taste and sight became sharper.
- Dreams became more vivid and colorful.

- Needed less sleep and slept deeply, waking up feeling rested.
- Became more aware of my true mission in life and my reason for living.
- Became calmer and more peaceful.
- Temper subsided.
- Stopped getting agitated.
- Gained greater spiritual awareness.
- Intuition became extremely keen.
- Relationships improved.
- Felt more love and compassion for all living things.
- Gained more flexibility.
- Gained more inner peace and contentment.
- Achieved complete joy and happiness.

Students ask me how long it took me to heal, and how long I think it will take them to heal. Everyone is different and in a different state of health. Everybody is unique and heals in his/her own way, and at his/her own pace. I do believe, however, that one reason I healed so quickly is because I did spiritual mind work and prayers, and that I had absolute total faith and belief that the Living Foods Lifestyle would heal me. I let go of all fear and doubt. I didn't try to second-guess the program. I took it on faith!

Also, I stuck to the program I've outlined in this book, eating and drinking the four main healing foods, green juices and watermelon juice almost exclusively for six months. I did eat some fresh fruit and vegetables that were not blended into the Energy Soup, such as celery, cucumbers and tomatoes. There were even times I "fell off the wagon" and ate something cooked, but each time I went right back to Living Foods. I found that when I ate something cooked I felt terrible. The healthier I became, the more cooked food disagreed with me.

My belief that the Living Foods Lifestyle would work for me was more powerful than the recipes I ate. I focused on the things I needed to do to get well, even when they weren't my favorite things to do. I repeatedly stepped out of my comfort zone to grow and heal. No matter how bad it seemed, I always related what I was going through to how I would've felt if I'd had surgery and taken chemotherapy.

When I thought of the alternative – nausea, hair loss, exhaustion, and who knows what else – eating this food and detoxing seemed mild in comparison. I counted my blessings every day, and gave thanks for the chance to heal in a non-invasive, non-toxic way. Every day I thank God for the opportunity to experience this powerful form of healing.

A DAY OF HEALING IN MY LIFE

People want to know what I do each day. They're curious about my routine, which includes food, exercise, and body, mind and spirit work. I suggest this routine to students as a foundation for healing. It may seem drastic, but it worked for me and I've seen it work time and time again for people with all types of health challenges, many of which have been critical. It takes discipline, but it's worth it.

After a few weeks of living this way, I created new habits that will stay with me for the rest of my life. It became easier the longer I did it. I continue to grow in my journey, and as I learn more, my eating and lifestyle become simpler. Fresh fruit, vegetables and greens are easy for me to find most anywhere in the world, and I feel great when I eat these foods.

- In addition to the healing foods I eat, I also meditate, pray and do spiritual mind treatments each day. I practice Bikram Yoga. The room is heated in this form of yoga, so I sweat and detox in the process. I used to go to the gym and train with weights, but I've found yoga has taken me to a new level of fitness I never experienced with weight training. With yoga I've improved my strength, endurance and stamina more effectively and quickly than pumping iron. Yoga also offers emotional and spiritual benefits. It accomplishes so much more than all other exercises I've tried, and it does it all at the same time! It is truly a meditation and exercise in one!
- I use my chi machine every day. It helps to detox, align and free up any energy blocks in my body. I love this little machine. It is wonderful to keep the energy freely moving throughout the body and it feels great on my back. There are many benefits to using the chi machine, and I highly recommend it.
- I get out in the sun every day for at least 30 minutes. As Ann Wigmore recommended, I sunbathe nude so I can receive the sun's rays over my entire body. I don't use sunscreen. Also, the pre-cancerous spots on my face have all healed. I thought they

came from sun damage, but I discovered they came from a toxic body and a dirty colon. When I cleaned up my body, the sores and spots healed. The sun is good for helping to dry up Candida. I usually get in the sun before 11:00 a.m. or after 3:00 p.m.

- I enjoy soaking in a tub filled with Epsom salts or Sea Salt and essential oils. This was especially beneficial when I was going through heavy detox. Sometimes my lower back and legs would ache, and soaking in a salt bath gave me instant relief and helped me rest. I use essential oils to help me continue healing. Special oils such as Ab-Ez, Let It Go, Living Well and No Plague are a part of my daily routine. These oils are designed to work on specific areas to open up, balance, clarify, detox and release.

- I schedule regular consegrity therapy and massage therapy sessions each week or so, and I know this has helped me heal and release toxins. The therapeutic touch during massage is soothing and healing to my body, mind and spirit.

- I do daily enemas and wheatgrass juice implants. In the beginning I did colonics twice a week, before cutting back to once a week, then every other week, then once a month. Now I have a colonic four times a year, at the change of each season.

- I go to a holistic chiropractor who uses bio-energetic synchronization technique (BEST), color therapy and flower essences.

- I walk my dog and get out in nature, remembering to breathe deeply. I love to commune with nature and now I can truly enjoy the outdoors because I am no longer plagued with allergies.

- I take the time to nurture myself, and I enjoy every moment! This is something I really had to work on because I tended to ignore my own needs and take care of everyone else. I now honor my spirit by taking the time to care for myself. Vacations and time off from work are important to me, and I make time for them. I get some of my best ideas when I don't have to think about work or other responsibilities – my mind is relaxed and open to endless possibilities. In my other jobs I skipped vacations because I was a workaholic. Eventually it caught up with me, making me even more tired and depressed. Now I realize everything will get done, and I don't drive myself as hard. This has been a wonderful gift, and I know it will help me live a longer and happier life.

MY DAILY ROUTINE

ENEMAS

I do an enema first thing in the morning. I've been doing them for a while so my colon is pretty clean. After an enema I implant 2 to 4 ounces of juiced wheatgrass into my colon. If your colon is extremely impacted, do two to four enema bags of reverse osmosis water to really cleanse the colon, then implant wheatgrass juice.

Always use good spring or filtered water such as reverse osmosis. The quality of the water going into your body is of the utmost importance. You can put a few blades of wheatgrass in your water and swish it around for a few minutes to help bring "life" to the water. While doing an enema, massage the colon to help release impacted fecal matter. Eliminate completely and repeat if necessary to get the colon as clean as possible before implanting wheatgrass juice.

Implant 2 to 4 ounces of wheatgrass juice in the colon and hold for 10 to 15 minutes. (Use a bulb syringe or a 2-ounce plastic plunge syringe, or put the wheatgrass juice in an enema bag. If you use an enema bag, put 6 ounces of wheatgrass in to compensate for what will be left in the bag because it won't all drain out.)

Implant 2 ounces of wheatgrass vaginally to help dissolve fibroids and other tumors, and to help with germs and bacteria.

While I'm doing my enema and implants I begin my spiritual work and prayers. This is a quiet time for me, and it's excellent for my time management. I'm always thinking about the healing I get from enemas, which helps me enjoy the experience rather than dread it.

Sometimes I do an enema and implant wheatgrass in the evening as well. During my first six months I did this faithfully, but for the most part now I only do morning enemas and implants. These things are important when you want to achieve the maximum results in the shortest time. The more serious you get with the four main healing foods, green juices, watermelon juice, enemas and wheatgrass implants, the faster you will heal.

EATING

This is an example of what I consumed each day during the first six months.

- 36 to 64 ounces of <u>Rejuvelac</u>.
- 36 to 64 ounces of <u>Energy Soup</u>.

- 8 to 16 ounces of Vege-Kraut.
- The above foods nourished me so well at the cellular level that I found I needed less and less food. If I was still hungry, however, I ate cucumbers, a salad of mixed baby greens and avocado, I made a raw salad dressing or used a little lemon juice and garlic.
- I ate crunchy vegetables such as zucchini, cucumbers and celery when I wanted something to chew.
- I ate lots of dark green, leafy vegetables such as kale and collards. I constantly had to remind myself to chew all food thoroughly. (I still do – not chewing my food well enough is a bad habit of mine.)
- I drank green juices and watermelon juice. One of my favorite green juice mixtures was – and still is – kale, cucumber, parsley and celery.
- At first I ate almost no fruit (because I had Candida) and stuck with the four main foods. Now, after being on the Living Foods Lifestyle for a while, I've simplified my life even further by eating more fruits, vegetables and greens. I can always find good organic fruit, which makes traveling easy. I don't make all the fancy recipes now like I did when I was first making the transition from cooked food to raw and Living Foods. I keep it simple!

Now that my tumors are healed, I've added a variety of other raw and Living Foods dishes to my daily menu, but I've found the simple foods are the ones my body likes and responds to best. When I keep it simple, I feel better. If I feel tired or get mucous after eating any food, I know that food is not the best for me. I'm spoiled now because I feel so good all the time. If I eat something that makes me feel less than my best, I take special note of it and avoid that food in the future. I finally understand that what I eat directly affects me. Even improperly combined raw and Living Foods, too many nuts, seeds and rich dishes can cause me to have digestion problems. Just because food isn't cooked doesn't necessarily mean it's good for you, especially in the wrong combinations.

As I was making the transition to raw and Living Foods, I cheated from time to time and ate some of the old cooked food recipes. I could immediately tell my body didn't like those recipes anymore. My body's unfavorable reaction to cooked food has encouraged me to stay on the Living Foods Lifestyle forever. If you fall off the program by eating something cooked, don't give up. Just go back to eating the good foods you know you need. We're all human, and most people, including me, are going to eat cooked food sometimes. In the beginning this was more of a problem for me, but now that I've been on the Lifestyle for some time, I don't really want cooked food. When my husband and I travel, or when we're celebrating a special occasion, I will occasionally eat something cooked, but I always feel tired afterward and I usually get mucous, gas and bloating. When that happens it reminds me once again how fortunate I am to have found this Lifestyle.

CHAPTER
THREE

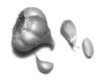

DISEASE AND OUR SOCIETY:
THE CAUSE IS IN OUR BODIES;
SO IS THE CURE

My true healing came about by making a total lifestyle change – not just following another fad diet. I can't stress this enough. Sometimes students come to my training classes thinking they'll learn a few recipes, make some changes in what they're eating, drink a couple of ounces of wheatgrass juice each day and, magically, they will heal. Unfortunately, there isn't any single magic recipe or drink that, by itself, can heal. It takes much more. True healing requires healing of the body, mind and spirit.

Because health is affected by so many things, it was important that I looked at my life in detail when I wanted to get well. Sometimes people ask me, "How did you do it?" They're hoping I'll give them a magic solution – tell them a few good things to eat, a couple of exercises to do, a book or two to read and that'll be it.

Students sometimes want the greatest results with the smallest amount of effort. That's typical of our society. We want a quick fix. That's why drugs are so popular. We think we can just pop a pill and take care of all our problems. Over time we have discovered that pills aren't the answer. Most people who take pills will tell you they don't like doing it, and if they could find something that worked better, they'd stop. I know I don't want to pop pills all day long. Some people who have come to me for help changing their lifestyles were taking handfuls of pills each day – everything from prescription drugs to synthetic vitamins and minerals. In almost every case each person told me taking pills wasn't the quality of life they had in mind. With the Living Foods Lifestyle I get my medicine, vitamins and minerals all from fresh live food – no more popping pills!

Think about this for a minute: If you have a headache and you take an aspirin, are you really getting rid of the headache? Of course not, you've only dulled or masked the pain with a drug. Did that fix anything? No! What will happen the next time you have a headache? Will you take more pills? How often do you have to get a headache before you begin putting two and two together? Did you get it because you ate too much sugar, preservatives, additives, colors, dyes and chemicals or because you're stressed out? To get well, we must understand what we're doing to make ourselves sick, and change those things. Doctors will never have all the answers. Many times they're stumped about what's really going on with their patients. They diagnose as best they can and prescribe a drug or surgery to "fix" the problem. Does it really "fix" it? When they cut out the cancer, do they get rid of all of it? Will it come back in another area of the body? Will we just keep removing parts of ourselves until there's nothing left to take? Will we keep taking so many drugs until we can't function anymore? How toxic will your body have to get before you wake up and do something about it? I let myself get completely out of control thinking I'd go on forever, never having to worry about the consequences of my actions, and then one day it caught up with me.

One reason I have such an aversion to pills is that for almost nine years I was married to a pharmacist. Our medicine cabinet contained every pill you could imagine. If I got a headache, he gave me a pill. If I had a stomachache or diarrhea, I took another pill. Sinus pills, diet pills, indigestion pills, aspirin, Tylenol, cough remedies and most prescription drugs were at my disposal. We had pills everywhere, but they never really fixed anything.

When I divorced I stopped taking prescription pills and began seeking a more natural way to care for myself. I saw a chiropractor and started taking new pills – vitamins and supplements. I hoped popping vitamin pills would bring perfect health, but it didn't. Taking vitamin pills to supplement all the dead food I was eating wasn't the answer. Still, over the years I spent thousands of dollars on the best vitamins money could buy.

I was so glad when I learned that with the Living Foods Lifestyle I would get my vitamins from my food and would no longer have to rely on buying expensive pills.

Not taking pills is just one way the Living Foods Lifestyle has changed and improved my life. I've seen it positively change the lives of hundreds of others, and I believe it will work for anyone who truly embraces it. Once again, this idea isn't new or new age – it's the oldest way of eating and living known to man. I believe it's the original way God intended us to live and eat. For thousands of years before the discovery of fire, we did live this way.

We read about people who lived hundreds of years during those early days. What did they know and do then that we don't know and do now? They had no vitamins or supplements. They ate simple, uncomplicated raw food – mostly fruit and wild plants. What happened along the way to get us off track? Why did we begin killing food and cooking it? What possessed us to eat dead, decaying animal flesh? Whatever it was, we have suffered much from our ignorance and practices.

I believe diseases are directly linked to the food we consume. It's no mystery! It amazes me that many doctors tell us what we eat doesn't affect our health. That's absurd. Everything we put in our bodies affects us, either positively or negatively. I wonder why doctors don't want to admit this. I've known teenagers with acne so bad their faces looked like pepperoni pizzas, which was probably exactly what they were eating. Some dermatologists tell them acne has nothing to do with the food they eat. Instead, they give them antibiotics and skin creams, then charge thousands of dollars for peels and potions. I don't wonder at the doctor's motivation to give them pills, powders, potions and treatments, do you? When the body is toxic and the toxins can't get out through normal channels such as the bowels, they seep out through the skin. If you want beautiful skin, clean the inside of your body – how you look on the outside is directly affected by how toxic you are inside.

CAUGHT ANYTHING LATELY?
TOXICITY & DEFICIENCY:
THE TRUE CAUSE OF DISEASE

Lots of people think they "catch" a cold or "catch" the flu. Can't you just picture us all, running down the street as fast as we can, chasing after a big, juicy cold or this year's flu bug? Oh yeah – I want to spend lots of time in that fun activity. We'll call it "The Great Cold and Flu Chase." We'll sign people up and ask them to get sponsors. We'll raise lots of money for cold and flu research. Sounds ridiculous, doesn't it? And just as ridiculous is the thought that we "catch" something like a cold or the flu.

Colds and other diseases aren't something we run after until we catch them. We get sick because there's an imbalance in our bodies. Allergies don't manifest because we are "allergic" to pollen, ragweed, goldenrod, dust, foods or any other outside substances. Allergies come from within the body because we're out of balance. I used to be plagued with allergies of every kind imaginable, but it was really myself I was allergic to. When I was young, my mother took me to the doctor for my allergies. They scratched my skin here and there, waiting to see if I'd have a reaction. I reacted to almost everything, and nothing the doctors ever did helped get rid of my allergies. Every year I suffered from sinus, hay fever and pollen allergies. My nose ran, my eyes watered, my throat felt scratchy. Nothing helped until I found the Living Foods Lifestyle. Once I cleaned up my system, all my "allergies" just "magically" went away. When the body is out of balance it reacts to outside stimulants, germs and viruses; the result is symptoms of distress we call allergies.

Diseases don't happen to us in an instant. Diseases result from years of neglect, imbalance, toxicity and deficiency in the body. You may be thinking, "What about a small baby who's sick, someone who hasn't had years of abuse and bad diet?" My answer is more questions, "What about the health of the father and the mother of that baby? How healthy were they when the baby was conceived? How nourished was the mother two to five years before conception of the baby? What did the mother eat during the pregnancy? Was the baby breast or bottle-fed?" All these things affect health. What the mother eats before and during pregnancy affects her baby. After the baby is born what she eats goes into her breast milk and is ingested by her baby. Many babies get off to an unhealthy start because of their parents' poor eating habits and poor health. If either parent smokes, a baby is likely to be sickly, have allergies and "catch" colds.

So, if we don't "catch" a cold or any other disease, what makes us sick? Many people think bacteria, germs and parasites are the culprits. In reality these so-called culprits are a part of the natural process. They come out of hiding, so to speak, when they have a job to do. Parasites perform a necessary function: cleaning up decaying matter, such as meat, within the body. After learning how meat rots in the colon – something I'll talk more about in Chapter 5 – many students decide to give up eating meat forever! When there's no rotting, putrefied food in your colon, parasites won't have to come out of hiding to do their job. Clean up the colon and clean out parasites.

Each organ and gland plays a special role in keeping the body working efficiently. The pancreas, for example, has a tough job to do when a person eats bad food. It produces digestive juices and enzymes so we can process the various elements in our food. When a person eats easy-to-digest Living Foods, the atoms and molecules are easily separated so they can be collected by the lymph system and used by the glands, cells and tissues. It's important to keep the pancreas operating at its optimum by making good food choices. The pancreas likes raw and Living Foods.

The body's glands – the pineal, thyroid, thymus, pancreas, adrenal and sex glands – function best when their cells are properly nourished with Living Foods. They can't function on cooked, dead food. Glands play an important part in our mental, emotional and spiritual health. When the glands become unbalanced from eating cooked, non-nutritious foods, symptoms abound. There's no limit to the misery these symptoms can bring, and they can change daily, even hourly, keeping you in a state of turmoil.

Nature is miraculous and perfect in the way it works. Take gardening, for instance; in a non-organic garden we spray chemicals and pesticides to get rid of the bugs, but in an organic garden pests stay away without the use of strong chemicals. A little cayenne pepper spray is even more effective at getting rid of bugs without using chemicals that are harmful to pets, as well as the human body. Pesticides, chemical fertilizers and other chemicals kill healthy microbes and earthworms, and contaminate crops at the same time. Nature, in all its intelligence, sends in bugs and insects to eat unhealthy crops, because Nature always demands that life evolve toward health. Our bodies are subject to these same conditions. When there is unhealthy, decaying matter in the body, disease is Nature's way of cleaning up. The way to get rid of disease from the body is to get rid of the cause of disease.

TREAT THE CAUSE, NOT THE SYMPTOMS

There's a difference between the cause of disease and symptoms. Treating symptoms will never "cure" a disease. Symptoms can change quickly and become difficult to treat. Drugs and surgery suppress symptoms and temporarily claim to "fix" the problem, but do nothing to get rid of the disease short of cutting or burning it out. In fact, the more drugs we take, the more the body becomes immune to drugs. You may already know that some antibiotics once used to "treat" disease no longer work because the body has become immune to them. The same is true for many other drugs – once they have been used to try to get rid of disease, the body becomes immune to them. When drugs don't work, disease returns with a vengeance. The body gets sick because it's toxic and enzyme deficient. If you want perfect health, you must remove toxicity and rebuild deficient enzymes.

Symptoms and disease are not the same things. Symptoms, in fact, are warnings that come from disease of long standing. There are so many different symptoms of the body that it would be impossible to keep up with all of them. I believe many symptoms start in the colon with improperly digested food. The colon becomes impacted with fecal waste, and the body becomes sick. The problem is that symptoms can jump around and change from moment to moment. That's why it's so important to address the real problem by changing our habits.

Treating symptoms will never solve health problems. In fact, treating symptoms with drugs can lead to more toxicity and deficiency and more symptoms and disease. Turning to drugs to fix our problems can cause a never-ending cycle of sickness. Many people take handfuls of drugs each day and are no better off. In fact, they may be worse off. Drugs are expensive and they don't really "cure" disease. At best they treat the symptoms. To heal your body, you must get to the cause and change the habits that created the problem. Treating symptoms is a never-ending battle, and one that will never cure you.

WONDER DRUGS DON'T WORK WONDERS

Our bodies try to tell us when something is wrong, but we ignore these warning symptoms. When we get heartburn, indigestion or acid reflux, we take a pill and hope it will go away. We keep eating the foods that cause these problems, and we go on hoping that by some miracle a drug will help us digest greasy, hot, spicy food with no adverse effects. Antacid manufacturers are making a fortune because we like to eat pepperoni pizza and chocolate cheesecake with Coca-Cola and cappuccino.

These "wonder drugs" may help a little, or maybe not at all. They may start out helping then quit. But we don't care; we just keep suffering because we don't want to give up our favorite foods, no matter how bad they make us feel. I used to keep Zantac, Pepcid AC, and Rolaids in my purse at all times, just to be sure all my bases were covered. Lying down was complete misery when I had severe heartburn and acid reflux. "Who cares, let's eat!" used to be my motto, but not anymore. Thank goodness I don't have any more acid reflux, heartburn or indigestion since adopting the Living Foods Lifestyle. After only a few days of Living Foods, all those problems disappeared.

Headaches are common among most people. I used to have a headache or two every week, sometimes for days in a row. Sometimes they were just annoying; often the pain stopped me dead in my tracks. From the slightest ache to the most severe migraine, we can trace symptoms back to stress, a toxic colon and bad foods. I used to think it was OK to take a pill to "fix" minor inconveniences such as headaches and indigestion. However, serious conditions such as heart disease, cancer, diabetes and high blood pressure are the result of letting little problems go unchecked. Learning that I must nourish my body properly to feel good and be disease-free was liberating. Symptoms were my body's way of screaming for help. It isn't natural to feel bad, but many people accept aches and pains as a part of life. Little symptoms that go ignored can lead to serious disease over time. Sooner or later, an out-of-balance lifestyle will catch up with us, and we will pay the price. The sooner we begin listening to our bodies and paying attention to their warnings, the sooner we can make changes that will help us experience the health we were intended to have.

When people get sick they turn to the doctor, hoping he or she will be able to fix everything. Doctors try to diagnose the problem, but because symptoms change from day to day – even moment to moment – this can be difficult. That's why so many people are taking handfuls of drugs. A drug intended to fix one problem can actually create another, leading to a never-ending cycle of more and more drugs. Drugs add to the body's toxicity, and instead of helping the problem, can actually make it worse. Drugs don't heal, they just treat symptoms, and they don't even do that well in most cases!

Most doctors are trained to treat symptoms related to disease. Many times they treat a patient with drugs and surgery, which may seem to work temporarily. In time, however, disease returns and you're back in a never-ending cycle of drugs and surgery. Is the answer cutting out body parts one after another until we're left with nothing? It's time to get serious about addressing the root of disease and correcting our lifestyle so we can change the outcome. Treating symptoms will never be the answer. Find out what you're doing to create your problem, and change it! If your food and lifestyle are out of control, your health will be too. You can decide to be healthy or sick. It's entirely up to you! Are you willing to make changes in what you do if it's really going to make you feel better?

If you always do what you've always done, you'll always get what you've always gotten. Make changes and get benefits!

ALLERGIC TO THE WORLD

I believe almost everyone who comes to me with health problems is suffering from some kind of allergy. Why? Allergies come from digestive disorders, and most people's digestive systems are weak and not functioning properly. This is because people eat so much cooked food. Cooked food has no enzymes to help digest it properly, so the body has to pull from its own supply of enzymes to digest it. When enzymes are taken from other parts of the body for use in digestion, the body begins to break down. When the body uses up its own supply of enzymes to replace missing enzymes in cooked food, disease begins. If the body isn't given proper nutrition through food, it becomes fatigued and allergic.

Even "health food," if not properly assimilated by the body, offers no benefits. Much so-called health food isn't healthy at all. It's processed, packaged and dead! Most people I work with have digestive problems and are not assimilating their nourishment. Many don't believe they have allergies because they think allergies have something to do with dust, pollen or a particular food. What they don't realize is that allergies are severe digestive problems that result from a lack of digestive enzymes. Their symptoms of allergies can be quite extensive.

Other causes for digestive problems include a breakdown of the immune system due to stress, pollution and food. Eating too fast and too much, and talking while eating, can also cause digestive problems. It's best to be quiet and relaxed while eating, and to only eat when you're hungry. Instead, most people are rushed when they eat and don't chew their food long enough before swallowing. Often, people with digestive problems are quite hungry. They eat large amounts of food, but they're really starving because of a lack of true nourishment. This overabundance of food rots in the body, causing numerous problems. The quickest way to restore the body and get rid of allergies is to eat raw and Living Foods that are full of enzymes.

Follow these guidelines to get the most from the foods you eat:

- First, relax before you eat and, if possible, eat in silence. Too much talking and socializing while eating can lead to eating too fast and eating too much.
- Overeating is hard on the body. Eat smaller amounts that the body can handle more easily.
- Don't eat too many different types of food at one time. The mono diet – one food at a time – is a great way to eat. It gives the body time to digest one food before putting more food in. Take it easy!
- Don't eat late. This is one of my own problems; I continually remind myself to eat my evening meal earlier. Allow the body three to four hours to digest food before going to sleep.
- Don't drink with your meal. Doing so dilutes digestive juices and makes it hard for the body to digest food. Wait two hours after eating before drinking.

FOOD ADDICTION: A FATAL ATTRACTION

Most people are addicted to something. Does that shock you? Probably not! Addictions are rampant and they range from alcohol and drugs to cigarettes and food. People can have hundreds of other addictions. I believe addictions are caused by deficiencies in the body, and the only way to restore the body is to give it good, nutritious Living Foods. When the body is deficient it craves the elements it's missing. I believe addictions can be treated successfully with the Living Foods Lifestyle.

I believe addiction to the wrong food is our number one health downfall. I am a food addict, so I can speak from my own experience. Does it surprise you that I would admit I'm addicted to cooked food? I'm actually addicted to eating, period! It's true, and it's been an important part of my healing to be able to admit that to myself. All my life I've eaten for the wrong reasons. I stuffed myself with creamy comfort foods and sugar to try to fill a void I felt within. I never thought about what I was eating and how it was affecting my health. I ate because I liked the way the candy bars and mashed potatoes tasted. They comforted me, but they didn't nourish me. What happened? I lost control, and I didn't know the truth about food.

What has happened to people eating to nourish, heal and rebuild their bodies? People rarely think about what food is really doing to their bodies. I never gave it a thought before I got sick. Most of us eat because it tastes good, with no regard for the nutritional benefits.

Are you eating to live, or living to eat? Food is for nourishment, healing and rebuilding the body. Think about what you eat, because you are what you eat!!

Before I put food in my mouth now, I think about what I'm eating and how it can help me. For the first time in my life, I eat to nourish and heal my body. The reward I get is a healthy body and enhanced energy. I can't tell you how happy I am to feel so good all the time. I feel free. Every day is a celebration. I'm no longer a prisoner of my own addictions.

FOOD ADDICTIONS ARE RAMPANT

You've already heard me say I personally think food addictions are the most serious of our addictions. No one gets put in jail for eating too much cheesecake or French fries. Unlike illegal drugs, cooked food is legal and so is overeating. Because we're addicted to the salt, sugar and grease in processed and cooked food, we don't want to give it up. We eat so much, and yet we get nothing that's of any use to our bodies. We're never satisfied because we're getting little or no nourishment to our cells.

I wonder how many people will die this year from smoking cigarettes? I wonder how many people will die from eating cooked food? Heart disease, diabetes, cancer – you name it – these "serious" diseases are directly linked to what we eat. The only way to give up a food addiction is to change the way you eat and the way you think about food. Replace food that's bad for you with food that's good for you. Learn to like new things with new tastes. Learn to eat for healing and nourishment and not out of addiction.

It's not easy to admit you're addicted to food. I never thought of myself as an addict until I began to cleanse my body with nourishing, energizing foods. I began to feel better and better, but cooked food still called my name. I thought about it. I dreamed about it. I wanted it. That's when I realized just how addicted I was.

Giving up an addiction can be difficult. That's why I recommend you get involved with a support group. You need a support system when you're making life changes or trying to give up bad habits. Books are great, but human support can make the difference between success and failure. Associate with people who will encourage you. During our monthly support group meetings students discuss their accomplishments and challenges. They see others facing the same challenges and each person is able to help others by sharing problems and crafting solutions. Students give each other hope and encouragement.

Like an alcoholic, a food addict is always recovering. Giving up bad food can be even harder than giving up alcohol. It's hard to avoid bad food. It's everywhere! Also, food gives us pleasure. We talk about "sinfully rich" dishes and indulging ourselves with chocolate as if the only reason we live is to eat. Eating has become the number one American hobby, pastime and escape. Everything we do seems to revolve around food. We have created a culture of food-addicted people. From the time our children are old enough to watch television they are sold sugar in many appealing forms. Cereals, cookies, cakes, candy bars and sodas all contain enormous amounts of sugar. Sugar is a drug, and it's poisoning adults and children everywhere. The addiction to sugar is rampant, and sugar kills.

I had a terrible sugar addiction when I went on the Living Foods Lifestyle. I felt I had to have something sweet after every meal. I overdosed on cookies and candy bars. I would go out in the middle of the night for a Baby Ruth candy bar. I didn't buy the small size either, I went for the king size, and I ate every bite in one sitting. I never thought I'd get to a point where I didn't crave sugar, but that's exactly what happened. After about six weeks of eating all raw and Living Foods I lost my sweet tooth. Now I can be around sweets and not have to eat them. I don't even want them anymore. I have no desire for sweets whatsoever. It's a miracle!

When we change what we eat, our tastes change. When we give our bodies healthy, nutritious raw and Living Foods, our bodies recognize this food and they're appreciative. When we eat raw and Living Foods we're nourishing our bodies on a cellular level. This is such a blessing for the body. Eating cooked food is one reason so many people are overweight. It's dead, with little or no nutritional value. We continue to eat because we're never nourished on a cellular level and we never feel satisfied. That means we're always hungry. I used to eat something sweet and then want something salty to get the sweet taste out of my mouth. No sooner had I consumed corn chips than I wanted Oreo cookies. After a half a bag of cookies, I'd get a taste for potato chips and onion dip. Then I'd want a double scoop of rocky road ice cream and so on. I call this my salty-sweet addiction. I'm so glad to finally be free of it!

A LOOK AT DISEASES AND THEIR CAUSES

HEART DISEASE

Do you know anyone with heart problems? What kind of food do they eat? Fatty, starchy foods are the main contributors to clogged arteries. When arteries are clogged, blood can't circulate throughout the body. Heart disease comes from toxicity and deficiency in the body. When people smoke, drink, take drugs and eat sweets, salt and fats, the body becomes toxic and blood vessels become clogged. The heart can't function properly with clogged arteries, and eventually it stops beating. I believe the Living Foods Lifestyle can restore the heart and prevent serious heart disease.

My father had his first heart attack at 42. All his life he ate rich food and drank alcohol. His family had a garden and a smokehouse. They ate meat and homemade biscuits and gravy. They grew a lot of vegetables in that wonderful garden, but they cooked those vegetables, sometimes for hours, until they were dead as a doornail. All those delicious kale and collard greens that could have been supplying enzymes, vitamins and minerals just went to waste because they were cooked to death.

"Cooked to death," now that's a mouthful. I never really thought much about that statement before I started the Living Foods Lifestyle. I had no idea that cooking my food was killing it, but it stands to reason now that I think about it. Fire destroys!

I see that between my father's poor eating habits and the unhappiness he felt about things that happened in his childhood and adult life, he created his own heart problems. He felt his mother never really loved him. He told me that throughout his life he always wanted his mother to tell him she loved him, but she never would. He told her he loved her again and again, but her only answer was, "Son, I think you do." That ate at him throughout his life and he was always "hungry" for love.

My father worked all his life in a textile mill. He took his first job there sweeping floors when he was only 16, and he worked his way up the ladder. When he was 41 he found out he was going to get the job he'd worked for all his life – head of the corduroy division. He'd actually been running the division for years waiting for his boss to retire. He planned the things he'd do with the extra money; how he'd provide more for his family, how we'd take bigger and better vacations, and build a bigger house.

One month before his promotion was to be official, the company announced it was planning to close his division. The leaders had decided corduroy would never catch on or make money. My father knew better. He said they were crazy to close the plant; that corduroy was the wave of the future. He was right, but it didn't matter. They closed the plant anyway. He was devastated, and he never recovered. He carried his anger and frustration with him until he died. First he developed heart problems, then diabetes and liver disease. One disease after another took over his body. Then he had a stroke.

My father was a wonderful man with much to give. Unfortunately he died far too young – at the age of 70. After years and years of disease, misery and sickness, he died an unhappy man. Food was one of his problems. But more than food, it was his thoughts that killed him. I wish I'd known about the Living Foods Lifestyle while he was alive so I could have helped him get well. I wish I could have helped him find the happiness he was so desperate for, but each of us is on our own path with our own lessons to learn and growth to experience. I loved my father and he knew it, but even that wasn't enough to make him happy. We are each responsible for finding our own happiness. No one can make someone else truly happy. Each person can only create happiness for himself or herself. If you know someone who's suffering with heart disease or any other sickness, tell him or her about the Living Foods Lifestyle. We do have a choice!

ASTHMA: HELP, I CAN'T BREATHE

Our lungs perform the important task of getting oxygen to our blood. Many people develop asthma and emphysema from bad habits, toxins and lack of enzymes. Our lungs try to work as best they can in the most unfavorable circumstances, with little nutrition and improper breathing techniques. Air is the most important element for energy. We get more energy from air than from food. We can go a few days or more without food, but we can't go even a few minutes without air. Air detoxifies and energizes the body.

Lung problems come from toxicity and deficiency in the body. Eating raw and Living Foods brings nourishment and oxygen to the blood and helps restore the lungs. If you know anyone who has damaged lungs from smoking or breathing bad air, tell them about the Living Foods Lifestyle. Fresh, Living Foods can help the lungs heal. My own family has been touched with these diseases and I know how devastating they can be. Many of my students with lung problems have experienced wonderful results through this marvelous way of living and eating. Wheatgrass juice is especially good for healing scars on the lungs, but it alone is not enough. Wheatgrass juice must be combined with raw and Living Foods to really work.

I'M SO DEPRESSED – GIVE ME PROZAC!

Nerve problems affect many people. Some try to tackle their problems by taking drugs. If we're sad and depressed, we take a pill, but pills will never solve this problem. The answer to nerve problems is to eat Living Foods. Nerve problems come from toxicity and deficiency in the body, just like every other disease. Nerve cells must have the right nourishment to function properly, and that begins with good raw and Living Food. Also, when the colon is impacted with fecal matter, nourishment can't be absorbed. The colon contains major nerve endings, so it's imperative to keep it clean and functioning properly. Proper colon cleansing is an important part of the Living Foods Lifestyle, and I will sing its praises again and again.

Millions of people suffer from depression. Are you one of them? Can you imagine the revenue antidepressant medications put in the drug companies' pockets? Billions of dollars are being spent on these medications. Drugs may seem to alleviate the problem, but depression can't be "cured" with pills. My depression went away after I was on Living Foods for only 10 days. My spirits lifted and my outlook on life improved dramatically. When we eat bad food, we're not properly nourished and we have little or no energy. This makes us feel depressed and unhappy. A toxic, deficient body is a depressed body.

Do you know any young children or teenagers who are on antidepressant medications? This is sad, because drugs will never fix this problem. Isn't it a shame that so many of our children are taking drugs? We give them drugs to calm them down and control their behavior. We give them drugs to lift their spirits. I believe that if parents changed their families' diets, we would see happy, healthy, energetic, well-adjusted children – not a bunch of kids on drugs. What message are we sending our children when we give them drugs for every ailment? Do you ever wonder why so many children turn to illegal drugs to make them feel better, to cope, or to fit in? Do we set this up by giving them drugs from the day they're born?

Rather than turning to drugs to solve the problem, let's turn to fresh, Living Foods, which give a natural high like no drug can. Take a look at the food the schools feed our children. It's horrible. Is junk food with no nutritional value supposed to nourish and energize our children? It's no wonder kids have so many health problems. Just look at what they're eating! Hamburgers, hot dogs, pizza, potato chips, carbonated sodas, ice cream, candy and popcorn do not nourish the body! What are we thinking? Oh yeah, I remember. The doctor says food doesn't affect the body, so it doesn't matter what our kids eat. Just give them what they want and keep them quiet. After all, when they get sick, there are always drugs. This is crazy thinking.

OH NO, I HAVE CANCER

Cancer has affected almost everyone these days, be it personal battles with the disease or those of friends and relatives. Almost everyone knows someone who has had, or still has, cancer. Cancer has become a scary reality to many people, and it's on the increase among our children too.

Many cancer patients come to the Living Foods Institute after receiving a "death sentence" from their doctor – just a few weeks, months or years left to live. Some come to the Institute only when they feel there's nowhere else to turn and they have nothing to lose. It's unfortunate that people will wait until it's almost too late to change their health. They put their faith in surgery and drugs and when that doesn't work they're desperate to try anything.

People who receive a cancer diagnosis are fearful. Doctors do a good job of scaring them to death by warning them that if they don't have surgery and chemotherapy they'll be dead in weeks, months or years. I've seen people try surgery and drugs, only to have the cancer return – be it months or years later. Chemotherapy weakens the body and makes it even harder to recover. Having surgery and taking drugs for disease must be an individual's decision, but so many tell me they wish they'd known about this Lifestyle before they took that route. If you know someone with cancer, tell him or her about the Living Foods Lifestyle so they can make a good decision for themselves. Cancer need not be a death sentence if a person is willing to make lifestyle changes.

Now they tell us there is a new miracle drug to "cure" cancer. It's too expensive for many people, but if you can afford it, it's supposedly your key to health. It's just one more drug added to the list. Is it the answer? If there's now a pill to cure cancer, what new disease will manifest next? As long as you eat cooked food, your body is going to get sick. Call it anything you want, cancer is just another disease caused by toxicity and deficiency in the body. Doctors might "cure" cancer, but there will always be another disease to strike people down. The Living Foods Lifestyle will detoxify and rebuild the whole person, inside and out, without drugs. Cancer is like any other disease; it comes from toxicity and deficiency in the body, mind and spirit.

It's extremely important that people who have already had surgery and taken chemotherapy for cancer nourish the body so it can detox and begin to heal. Sometimes, when people come to the Living Foods Institute they have already tried the surgery/drug route and they realize their bodies are now very weak. Living Foods can help restore energy and rebuild health in these people too. No matter what healing route a person has decided to follow, good basic nutrition is a key factor in health and healing. I didn't personally choose surgery and drugs, but I work with many who have. I welcome the opportunity to help everyone, no matter what their decisions about surgery and drugs have been in the past. It's never too late to restore health when there's a true willingness to change and a belief that the changes will work.

WHY AM I SO TIRED?

Boy, are we tired! We've created fancy names for our fatigue such as Chronic Fatigue Syndrome, Yuppie Flu, Epstein-Barr Syndrome and Fibromyalgia. I guess we think this sounds more glamorous than just saying we're tired and worn out. The simple fact is that most people can hardly make it through the day half awake. We become fatigued when our bodies are toxic and deficient, so it's no surprise we're dragging around, sleeping at our desks, and never have enough energy to even take a walk or do household chores. Many people's bodies hurt all over and it's getting worse with all the cooked, processed, denatured foods they're eating. Their bodies, starved for real nourishment, are rebelling. Did you know that about 90 percent of the food an average American eats is processed and devoid of any kind of nourishment?

Chronic Fatigue Syndrome and Fibromyalgia are directly related to toxicity and deficiency, especially enzyme deficiencies. When you eat dead foods you feel dead! Eat Living Foods and feel alive. Do you have plenty of energy from the time you get up until you go to bed at night, or do you barely slide along feeling like even the smallest task takes major effort? I used to want to sleep 8, 10 or 12 hours a night. Now, I bounce out of bed after only 4 to 6 hours of sleep, raring to go. No more naps after lunch or falling asleep before the sun goes down for me – I have to make myself stop and go to bed. I'm so full of energy and having so much fun doing all I do that I don't want to waste time sleeping. Low energy and fatigue come from toxicity and deficiency in the body. When you eat right, you feel great.

CANDIDA AND PARASITES DO WHAT TO ME?

If your childhood was anything like mine, you remember taking antibiotics, cough medicines and aspirin on a regular basis. We were vaccinated against everything from polio to measles. Those first antibiotics began destroying beneficial bacteria in our intestinal tract and colon, and yeast started to take over. As a result of taking antibiotics, millions of people today have developed a condition known as Candidiasis (Candida), an overgrowth of yeast. Birth control pills are another common cause of Candidiasis.

Candidiasis is serious. It causes symptoms ranging from yeast infections to fatigue, brain fog and depression. Most of my students have had Candida. I had it, and I didn't even know it. In fact, I didn't even know what Candida was. I never had one of the vaginal yeast infections that plague so many women, so I was surprised to find I had Candida. Do you know children plagued with ear infections? I had problems with my ears all my life. What I didn't know was that my ear infections were caused by yeast. When I adopted the Living Foods Lifestyle, my yeast problem went away. I tried other programs to eliminate yeast and got some results, but couldn't get rid of Candida until I was on the Living Foods Lifestyle for four months.

Many people are also plagued with parasites. When the body is toxic and deficient, and the colon is full of impacted, putrefied fecal waste, parasites multiply. These same parasites are sucking the life out of those who are infested with them. No one likes to talk about parasites and worms. It's disgusting to think our bodies might be full of them, but it's true. Candida and parasites were just two of the many problems that plagued me before I began the Living Foods Lifestyle. After just a few months on Living Foods, all my Candida and parasites were no longer a problem. What a relief!

HYPOGLYCEMIA: JUST TOO SWEET

More than 80 percent of all people are affected by hypoglycemia, and most don't even know it. The symptoms can manifest in many forms including depression, confusion, mood swings, cravings for sweets, fatigue, oversleeping, insomnia, blurred vision and just plain not feeling good. Some people begin to have symptoms of hypoglycemia after they have eaten sweets for a long time. Too much sugar in the mainstream American diet is a big problem. We're addicted to sugar and we crave it. Hypoglycemia is just one of the many problems created and aggravated by sugar. I was finally able to overcome my addiction to sweets after being on the Living Foods Lifestyle for about two months. I am so glad I don't crave sweets the way I once did.

In the body, the adrenal glands monitor the availability of sugar to the bloodstream and cells. When the adrenals are functioning normally, they secrete the appropriate amount of adrenalin to raise blood sugar levels as required. Metabolic processes and sugar levels get out of balance when adrenal glands aren't functioning properly. After years of eating processed, chemically treated, cooked foods, the adrenal glands become diseased. The adrenal glands would never fail and hypoglycemia wouldn't be a problem if we were continuously eating easy-to-digest, raw and Living Foods.

OBESITY – JUST ANOTHER WORD FOR FAT

So many people have come to the Living Foods Institute to lose weight. I hear time and again about the agony people go through because they are overweight. Obesity is about much more than just being fat. Obesity affects overall health and impacts a person psychologically. When I was overweight I thought about it all the time. I couldn't get it off my mind. If I saw a slender person, I envied them and longed to be like them. If I saw a fat person, I compared how fat they were to how fat I was. I felt better if they were fatter than I was. I thought about food all the time, too.

Now it seems as though I ate all the time and could never get satisfied. Food courts at the mall were pure torture. Between French fries and chocolate chip cookies, my visits became a feeding frenzy. I could hardly finish one food without thinking about the next. As a result, my weight continued to rise. My size 12 clothes became 14, then 16 and then 18. When I went to the doctor in February 1999 I was fast approaching size 20. I had to shop in the plus size sections and large women's stores, and they never had the fashions I wanted to wear. All my pants had elastic waists and I only wore oversize tops. I did everything I could to hide my body, and I hated to go anywhere because I was so self-conscious. I felt like a prisoner in my own body.

I realize now that my own unhappiness caused me to eat

so much. I had been carrying around anger and guilt for things that happened in my past. The more I ate, the less I had to deal with my feelings. I put on weight to insulate me from the world and my own feelings of sadness. Part of my healing was getting in touch with my feelings and letting go of old emotions that were holding me back. After working with so many people, I've come to realize that our emotions make us sick, and it's most important to acknowledge our feelings, forgive ourselves and others, release and let go if we want to move forward and truly heal. It was liberating to lose so much weight on the Living Foods Lifestyle, and even more liberating to lose the anger.

I wasn't expecting the weight to come off so easily, but to my pleasant surprise it almost seemed effortless. It was easier to lose the weight than the anger. I had been in denial for so long and I did not think I was an angry person, but situations frequently presented themselves that brought out anger in me. I had to finally look at that and to recognize where it was coming from. The Living Foods Lifestyle has helped me to get in touch with my true feelings and emotions. I have uncovered deep hidden "stuff" and I have healed and released it. It feels good to be free of the weight and the burdens I carried for so long.

If you want to see fat melt away, eat raw and Living Foods. If you stick to it, you will never have a weight problem again. As long as I ate raw and Living Foods I felt nourished and satisfied and the pounds melted away. I never felt hungry or like I was starving myself to death on Living Foods. As the pounds came off, I felt better and better. My energy level went up and so did my self-esteem. I cannot sing the praises of this Lifestyle enough when it comes to weight loss.

However, those people who are already thin or who have lost a lot a weight because of an illness need not despair. You can put on weight with the Living Foods Lifestyle just as you can take it off. It's all about proper food combining and exercise. I've helped AIDS and cancer patients gain 10 to 50 pounds or more with the Living Foods Lifestyle. The beautiful thing about it is that the body will get to its ideal weight with good health practices.

OH, MY ACHING FEET:
HIGH-HEELED SHOES AND OTHER BAD HABITS

High-heeled shoes should be outlawed! I almost ruined my feet wearing high heels, and my posture and organs suffered too. I know women who have worn high heels for so long that it's painful for them to stand flat-footed. The wrong shoes can not only ruin your feet, they can ruin your health. We should all take our shoes off more often and go barefoot. Our feet need fresh air.

High-heeled shoes are just one of many harmful habits we have developed. What habits of yours are affecting your health? Many people have muscle problems because their nerves and cells aren't functioning properly. This is because they follow the poor eating habits our society has adopted. Without proper fuel for growth and maintenance, muscles can't be strong. When we eat cooked, processed, chemically treated food, we aren't giving the body proper ingredients to produce superior fuel. When the body doesn't have proper fuel, it can't make muscle or support muscle strength. This causes aches and pains.

Little or no exercise also contributes to many aches and pains. All bodies need to be stretched and exercised. Get off the couch and go out for a walk. Lift weights. Take yoga. Move and breathe and give your body what it needs to flourish. If we feel bad, it's because we've done things to make ourselves feel bad. If we want to feel better, we have to do things that will help us feel better. Each person is completely responsible for his or her own health or illness.

IS DISEASE OVERTAKING THE WORLD?

There are many more symptoms and diseases plaguing society than those I have mentioned here, and new ones are cropping up every day. It doesn't matter what label you place on disease and symptoms, all come from the same two sources – toxicity and deficiency. Usually when a person is sick, he or she has been eating lots of cooked food. It's ironic that we can eat lots of food and literally starve ourselves to death because we're not getting the enzymes and nourishment we need to ensure health and life.

To make changes in our health, we must make changes in our lifestyle. We can choose to change and get well or choose to do nothing and get sicker and sicker. Even if a doctor has given a patient a "death sentence," it is never to late to make changes in order to regain health. I've worked with many people who've been given absolutely no hope by their doctors. Instead of accepting that diagnosis, they decide to make changes in their lives. As a result, they get well.

Through all my work with sick people and after having been sick myself, I know the root cause of disease is toxicity and deficiency. These conditions result from eating denatured, processed and cooked food. It's important to eat for nourishment and not just for the taste of food. When we eat food full of live enzymes we help our bodies restore health. We don't have to accept symptoms and disease. We can make changes if we really want to be healthy! It's completely up to us.

EVEN OUR PLANET IS SICK

Our planet is getting sicker every day. People are dying from more serious diseases at younger ages than ever before. Children take more drugs today than at any time in history. From a very early age most of us begin to accumulate toxins in our bodies.

You've already heard me talk about this and I'll say it again – one of the ways we do this is by taking drugs. Our parents and doctors gave us drugs and vaccines when we were kids, and now we give them to our own children. Our parents may have been – and we may be – well meaning, but drugs are toxic substances, and every time we take them ourselves or administer them to our children, we are contributing to the body's toxicity. Are doctors and parents supporting drug addictions by giving children prescription drugs? What are we teaching our children by the drugs that we give them for colds, flu and stomach aches? Does this give them the idea that drugs are OK? Where do we draw the line between good and bad drugs? Do we think that because it's a drug we can get by prescription, it's good, but if it's illegal and we can go to jail for using it, then it's bad?

Have you noticed how many drugs are advertised on television today? There's a major campaign to get us to take more drugs. I cringe every time I see those ads. First they tell us the name of these "wonder" drugs and then they tell us about the potential side effects: nausea, headache, liver problems, kidney problems, sexual side effects and so on. How are these drugs supposed to help us? Some side effects sound worse than the illness itself. What will kill us – the disease, or the drugs we take to cure it? The only way to heal our planet is to heal ourselves one person at a time. Only by taking full responsibility for your health can you help heal the world. You don't have to be sick. You can be well and healthy if you will take responsibility for doing the right things. The Living Foods Lifestyle can help each of us heal, and as a result it will help our world heal.

911 WAKE UP! WAKE UP!! WAKE UP!!!
EAT RAW AND LIVING FOODS AND BRING PEACE TO THE PLANET

Before September 11, 2001 I believed eating a raw and Living Foods diet was the best way to restore and maintain health. I've taught hundreds of people how to use the Living Foods Lifestyle to achieve total and perfect health. Now more than ever I'm convinced this is the only way to go if we are to achieve peace throughout the world. It has now moved beyond gaining our own health back, it has become paramount in gaining back the health and the peace of our world.

I believe the consumption of dead animal flesh, sugar, cooked and processed foods is a major contributor to anger, hostility and war in the world. I believe one of the reasons so many of our children are diagnosed with attention deficit disorder, depression and a host of other childhood diseases is the denatured, processed and cooked, dead food they're eating. I believe we're sicker than we've ever been in the history of the world, and it's getting worse every day. We must make changes now if we're to continue to live on this planet. Our past decisions have created our current problems. Every cause has an effect, and the effect of eating cooked, dead food is devastating disease and chaos throughout the world.

Not only is it important to eat nutritious raw and Living Foods for health reasons, now those reasons go even deeper. It's imperative that we reconnect with our true, spiritual nature, and the way to do this is by putting enzyme-rich raw and Living Foods into our bodies. When we eat these nutritious foods we do more than nourish our bodies, we nourish our spirits as well. Enzymes are the intangible life force that connects us with our true spiritual nature.

After I became a Living Foodist I noticed that I was no longer quick to anger, that my road rage disappeared and that things that had once bothered me began to roll off my back. I became more loving and gentle toward all people, animals and plants. I became more aware of my connection to all life and how we are all created from one spiritual energy. I began to realize even more than ever that I am a spiritual being temporarily inhabiting a human body. My compassion for others increased and my understanding of my purpose for living was revealed.

I've taught many others who have also reported the same changes in their own feelings and understandings of the truth. I realize eating a raw and Living Foods diet creates peace, love and harmony within and among all people. The Living Foods Lifestyle creates good karma.

Karma is made up of all the things we have done and all the things we have not done throughout our existence. Our karma is what we really are, at our core. Each of our lives is a direct reflection of what we truly believe and who we truly are. What goes around comes around, and as we kill animals and eat dead flesh, we create negative vibrations within ourselves. Consequently we create negativity in our world.

All of creation is connected. We're connected to animals, plants and to each other. As we've become callous about killing and eating animals, we've seen some people become callous about killing one another. Our world has gone crazy and we're all contributors to the insanity. We've lost our minds as we've lost our integrity. Where is the value of life? When will we take responsibility for the world we have created? How long can man continue to go through life with no regard for other lives? When our mentality centers on killing, we bring about our own death.

There are karmic consequences for eating dead animal flesh. Not only are the animals turning against us with diseases like "mad cow disease"; we are turning against one another with "mad people disease." The low vibration of cooked, dead animal flesh and other cooked foods has created a low vibration in human beings that translates into low vibrational thinking and actions. Thinking about killing people in order to gain peace is crazy thinking, and it does not come from those who are vibrating at a high spiritual level. Feelings of death and destruction come from a very low vibration. How does that happen? It happens when our minds and our thinking become clouded with toxins and poisons. Some of this comes from our thoughts and some comes directly from the food we eat.

Food does have a direct relationship on how you look, feel, think and react. Put Living Foods into your body and your thoughts turn to life and living. Put cooked, dead foods – especially dead animal flesh – and sugar in your body, and your thoughts turn to anger, agitation, conflict, war, disease and death. Why isn't more emphasis put on helping people change their way of living and what they're eating so we can change the world we live in? Have we moved so far away from the truth that we've completely lost touch with the significance food has in our lives?

Food was created to nourish and heal the body. Food was intended to be our medicine, but more and more we have turned to drugs and unnatural forms of "healing." We've polluted our bodies, minds and spirits with bad food, drugs and toxic thoughts, and we've created our own nightmare. Now, when we get a growth, a tumor or a cancer the first thing most people think about – and are told to do – is surgery. Cut the tumor out and take poisonous drugs to "kill" the bad cells. It's unfortunate that we've moved so far off track that we could even think such an idea. How in the world can we think that cutting something out of the body and then bombarding it with poisonous drugs could be a good thing? Where are our inner voices? Are we listening to the great intelligence that resides within each of us, or are we ignoring what it's telling us?

It's time we all wake up and detoxify our bodies and our minds of the substances and thoughts that have been making us and our world sick. Everything happens for a reason. Whatever the reason is that we've created and attracted the negative conditions we're living in, it's now up to us to change our thoughts and patterns – and to change our world into a better, more peaceful and loving place.

You can make a difference. You can do your part to help to bring peace to the planet. How, you ask? Take responsibility for your own decisions and your own health. When just one person begins to eat a raw and Living Foods diet, that one person becomes a more peaceful and loving individual. That loving energy reaches out to and influences other people. Soon there are two people eating raw and Living Foods, and as those two become more loving and peaceful they multiply to four. Feeling good and being healthy is something everyone wants and few really have. As each Living Foodist helps create another Living Foodist, we begin to heal the world one person at a time.

This is an idea whose time has come and nothing can stop it. Living Foods is not a fad! Living Foods will not pass by quickly in the night and be gone! Living Foods will bring total and perfect health! Living Foods is alive and growing! We must all spread the word. We must tell everyone, everywhere so they, too, can begin to eat Living Foods. As we change our own lifestyles we change the world.

We must all stand tall and proud and live in a world without fear. My husband and I have been on many airplanes since September 11, 2001. We've flown both inside and outside the country. Everything has gone with ease. The changes that have taken place in the airports, and in every facet of our lives, have caused us to pay attention. It may take a little more time when you travel, but that's no reason to stop. Fear isn't a good reason either. Fear paralyzes. Fear sickens. Fear debilitates. I have not felt fear during any of these global changes. I've continued to live my life as usual – full and exciting. I will not stop traveling. I will travel more than ever. I will enjoy this wonderful life with every experience and opportunity it brings. I will not be afraid. I believe that the Living Foods Lifestyle is why I feel this way. I know that everything is in Divine Order and that good will come from every experience.

All of us can unite in our mission to bring peace to the planet. We can agree to support each other to eat raw and Living Foods, and we will benefit from the peaceful and loving feelings that will come over all of us. We needn't stand idly by waiting to see what happens next, or to live in fear that something will happen. We can become proactive in creating our own world of peace and love. Peace is possible and it all begins with each of us.

We create our own reality with our individual thinking as well as our collective consciousness. We can manifest exactly what we want by thinking about, speaking out loud and writing down what we want. We create our world with our thoughts and our actions. Please take responsibility for your health. Please make changes in what you eat to supply your body with the enzymes and nutrition it must have to live healthy and disease-free. Please love yourself enough to use your willpower and exercise restraint in your eating habits. Give yourself the greatest gift you could ever give, the freedom and happiness of total and perfect health of the body, mind and spirit. Make a real difference in the world. Eat raw and Living Foods!

The September 11th incident happened on the fourth day of our monthly 10-Day Training Program. The phone began ringing with students wondering if we would still have class. We assured the students that all classes would be held and everyone showed up as usual. Rather than our covering the material as we usually did on Day

4, we shared our feelings about what had happened. These students had only been eating raw and Living Foods for four days and already they were experiencing great changes. As we shared, I heard time and time again from students that they hoped that we would be able to resolve this conflict peacefully. We prayed for world peace and Golden Keyed the situation, a process you'll learn more about in Chapter Five. We're doing something to change the world when we do something to change ourselves.

HEALING: CAN LIVING FOODS WORK FOR ME?

LET FOOD BE YOUR MEDICINE

Hippocrates, the ancient Greek physician known as the father of medicine, once said, "Let food be your medicine, let medicine be your food." This is a lesson each of us will benefit from if we practice it. I can't tell you how out of touch I was with the real purpose of food. I didn't understand the importance of what I ate until I got sick. Food was everything to me except medicine. I was living to eat, not eating to live.

God has given us every food we need to perfectly nourish our bodies. These foods are simple, fresh, organic and raw, not processed, genetically altered or cooked. When was the last time you ate pure, simple food? As a society, we're far away from the real reasons we should eat – to nourish and heal.

Today most people eat for every other reason imaginable. We eat because we're bored, depressed, happy, anxious, tired, lonely, frustrated, celebrating, mourning or just because the food is in the refrigerator. Many of us are addicted to cooked food and the way it tastes. I'm one of these people. I never realized how addicted I was until I began trying to give it up. I ate for every reason from depression to boredom. I ate when I was happy and when I was sad. I ate out of loneliness and just because I knew food was in the house. Cookies and ice cream would call my name, and instead of a cookie or two, I'd eat the entire bag. Instead of a scoop of ice cream, I'd eat two or three bowls. Talk about an addiction that's a killer – this one's both legal and lethal all in one.

Foods with sugar and fat comforted me, but they were also killing me. I had to get back to the original laws of nature and eat to restore my energy, health and vitality. Raw and Living Foods give me the most energy and vitality I can get anywhere. A pill, powder or potion will never give you the perfect health you desire. Only by making changes in your lifestyle will you attain health. Drugs don't fix anything! They may treat the symptoms, but they don't get to the root cause of why we got sick in the first place. Unless and until we address the cause of our diseases, we will continue to get sicker. At best, a drug can only temporarily mask the problem. I forgot pills, and let my food become my medicine. This is so easy! Don't complicate a perfect plan for health by trying to fix diseases with drugs. Change what you eat, and change your health. Change what you think, and change your world.

Health can be restored. I am not a doctor and I cannot recommend surgery or drugs. I can only speak for myself in saying that I wouldn't do either. I've been asked if everyone that follows the Living Foods Lifestyle heals. The answer is no. Healing is unique to each individual and depends on many factors, especially the person's attitude. In a few cases, people are so depleted from surgery and drugs – and from waiting so long to come to us – that there is little hope. However, I always encourage everyone to try it. What do you have to lose? Nothing! And you have everything to gain. In the majority of cases it's never too late as long as a person is willing to make the necessary changes and they truly believe it will work.

The human body is miraculous. It keeps on going in spite of the abuse it takes. The human spirit is even more tenacious. I have seen people so sick they could hardly walk into our Center. Some even had to be carried in. They were scared they might never get well. Then they began to change their thoughts and habits. They learned to expect health and to embrace the Living Foods Lifestyle. They experienced a complete body-mind-spirit cleansing and a rebuilding of their total selves. Then they "miraculously" got well.

Is it a miracle that the body, mind and spirit react to our doing the right things to maintain health? Or is it just common sense that if we take responsibility for our health and make the right choices in our lives, we'll be rewarded with good health, happiness and prosperity? Time and again people are reclaiming their power and restoring their health by eating the right foods, thinking the right thoughts, exercising, breathing properly and having faith that they are healed.

LIVING FOODS 101

There was so much I didn't know when I began my healing journey. Hundreds of questions ran through my mind. There was so much to learn – I didn't know where to begin. I asked many questions: "What is an enzyme? Why do I need them so much? What is a colonic? Does it hurt? Why should I do enemas and wheatgrass implants every day? Why can't I cook food? Do I have to eat everything raw for the rest of my life? Does this mean I'll become a rabbit and eat nothing but salads at every meal?" I was in a panic! Maybe you have the same questions and fears. Don't worry; it's not as complicated as you might think. In fact, it's easy. Let's start with enzymes.

THE IMPORTANCE OF ENZYMES

I can't overemphasize how important enzymes are to our health. Enzymes contribute directly to digestion, and without good digestion we don't get nourishment from the food we eat. We won't live long without enzymes. We can't conceive without enzymes, therefore the existence of future generations directly depends on enzymes. Enzymes are the catalysts that make cells function effectively. They make life possible by repairing and building the body. Enzymes are an intangible life force that directly connect us to our true spirituality. Our bodies require enzymes for every single activity. When we are in a healthy balance, our body manufactures the enzymes that fight infection and digest food. Enzymes make the liver, kidneys, lungs and every other organ function. Our hearts won't beat, we can't blink our eyes, and we won't lose or gain a pound without enzymes. Enzymes work non-stop to help keep our bodies in balance.

Enzymes are in every raw and Living Food we eat, and they help us digest each of these foods. Yet as important as they are to our survival, **we kill every single enzyme in our food when we cook it.** We destroy the very thing we must have to live and thrive on, before we can even get it in our bodies. Heating food to more than 105 degrees breaks down and kills the enzymes. This holds true for steaming or waterless cooking too – anything higher than 105 degrees, and the food is dead.

ENZYMES AND BODY WEIGHT

I've had weight problems all my life. Until now, weight has been a constant challenge. I've been consumed with thoughts of food – what to eat, what not to eat, how much of this, how little of that. I've starved myself on numerous occasions just trying to lose a few pounds. If only I'd known about enzymes before, I could've saved myself a lot of worry over my weight.

Cooked food is devoid of enzymes, so when we eat cooked food we only assimilate a small amount of it. We're starving our bodies on a cellular level with cooked food, so we tend to eat more and more. We're hungry all the time, and we're never satisfied. Begin eating raw and Living Foods and feel the difference in your body when you're being nourished on a cellular level. Suddenly you're not as hungry as you once were. Your energy levels increase and your metabolism balances. You will begin to feel satisfied when you eat, and you won't want processed or cooked food as much. The more you eat Living Foods, the more you'll want to eat them.

Enzymes also play an important part in gaining weight. I've worked with many people who, because of serious diseases, have lost large amounts of weight. Once they begin to eat Living Foods in a balanced diet, the body is restored and so is the weight. I've seen people gain 20 to 50 pounds or more by eating raw and Living Foods. So whether you need to lose or gain weight, the Living Foods Lifestyle can help you do it! It's all a matter of which foods you eat and in which combinations. By learning more about "real" food, you'll be able to make the right choices to achieve any result you want.

COOK IT, KILL IT!

Whether you eat meat or vegetables, remember – when you cook food, you kill it. When we stop cooking and learn new ways to prepare delicious, nutritious, enzyme-rich foods, we help our bodies return to perfect health. If you want your food warm, you can slightly warm it without destroying the enzymes. Just be sure you keep the temperature less than 105 degrees. Cooking, in addition to destroying all the enzymes, also destroys much of the food's nutritional value. You only get a small percentage of the original nutrition intended from cooked food, as opposed to the 100 percent nutrition you could get by eating your food raw. Raw food is full of vitamins and minerals; cooking destroys most of these elements.

Raw and Living Foods don't have to be boring; they can be delicious as well as nutritious. I was a gourmet cook before I began the Living Foods Lifestyle. I worried about what my friends and family would say when they found out I wasn't cooking anymore. I decided there was no reason for me to stop preparing fabulous food; I would just have to do it without cooking. I love to create gourmet Living Foods recipes. Preparing food without cooking is fun and easy. I save time, energy and money while healing my body and increasing my energy. People rave about my food now, and the bowls are practically licked clean at parties. I never talk about how healthy my recipes are; I just put them on the table and watch people feast. The quickest way to turn some people off is to harp on how Living Foods is the only way to go. I've found it's better not to say too much. People notice the positive changes and they want the same results. Actions speak louder than words. The best way to lead is by setting a good example.

Sometimes my students get so excited when they learn about the Living Foods Lifestyle they want to convert everyone, especially friends and family members. The problem comes when others are not ready to make a change and feel they're being pushed too hard. I've found the best approach to sharing information about Living Foods is subtlety. Coming on too strong can really turn people off. Remember that everyone is on his or her own individual path, and the only mind you can change is your own. If you're going to practice the Living Foods Lifestyle, do it for yourself, because you want to, not because someone else has tried to push you into it. When you do it for the right reasons, you'll be more likely to stick with it. As you make positive changes, your friends and family will notice. This is one of the best ways to win them over. When others see you glowing and healthy, they'll want what you have.

LIVING FOODS VS. RAW FOODS – WHAT'S THE DIFFERENCE?

Even though we use lots of raw food, this is the "Living Foods Lifestyle," not the raw food lifestyle. Let's talk about the difference in raw and Living Foods. Raw foods are those picked off trees or vines, such as apples, cucumbers, avocados, squash, tomatoes and bananas. Living Foods are beans, grains, nuts, seeds and berries that have been soaked and sprouted. When the sprout comes out of the grain, seed or berry it becomes a "Living Food," full of life and increased nutritional value. Ann Wigmore made the point about this being the Living Foods Lifestyle. She believed, as do I, that sprouted, Living Foods have a high nutritional value and can help restore health quickly. The vital energy springing forth in them as they sprout provides extra, super-charged energy.

Though we use many organic, raw fruits and vegetables in our Living Foods recipes, we believe those recipes with sprouted, Living Foods are the real powerhouses. We soak and/or sprout every nut, seed and berry before we use it in a recipe. This fresh, live nutrition brings us back in touch with nature, back to our original roots, back to the real reason we should eat – for health, nutrition and rebuilding the body.

Try this experiment: If you have a baby, or know someone who does, place cooked and raw food on the same plate and offer it to the baby. The baby will choose the raw food every time! Even babies know what's best for them to eat. I used to crave cooked food all the time; now I love the taste of fresh, raw food. It just took a little time for my body to adjust to the new tastes of raw and Living Foods. Now there's nothing more refreshing and satisfying to me than cool cucumbers or fresh, ripe avocados.

I remember thinking food had to have a sauce, dressing or gravy to taste good. Now I get pleasure from simplicity. I enjoy the taste of fruits and vegetables with nothing on them. I've simplified my life and my eating habits. When I was transitioning off cooked food, I ate the more fancy raw dishes. They reminded me of the rich, cooked food I was used to. Now that I've been eating raw and Living Foods for a while, I no longer crave those fancy dishes. I enjoy real, fresh, alive, simple, unprocessed foods that are ORGANIC, of course!

On the final day of every 10-Day Training, we throw a party. Graduating students can invite friends, family and business associates to an incredible feast with a wonderful array of delicious Living Foods. At some of the first parties I would pile my plate high with raw lasagna, vege-paté, candy truffles, fiesto crackers and every other delicious treat on the table. As time passed and I became healthier, I noticed I didn't want the rich gourmet dishes anymore. I just wanted simple fruits and vegetables. Now that's all I eat. Even when we have the party, I have no desire to eat fancy foods. For me, simpler food is better. Listen to your body as it changes. What might be good at one stage may not be suitable at another. Trust yourself and follow your inner guidance.

THE LIVING FOODS LIFESTYLE IS ABOUT ABUNDANCE

You might think the Living Foods Lifestyle sounds restrictive, but let me assure you, it's not. You won't have to live on salads the rest of your life. You can have a life full of food adventures. You'll discover – perhaps for the first time – what real, fresh food tastes like. You'll experience a delicious variety of flavors and combinations. The creamy, exotic taste of the durian may excite your taste buds. The refreshing simplicity of a cucumber may satisfy your desire. Keep it simple – just wash it and eat it. Zucchini, celery and tomatoes will be at your beck and call, or you can opt for lasagna or yam pie with macadamia date cream. You can indulge your passion for food and go way beyond where you've gone before with your taste and your health. You won't give up good-tasting, wonderful foods; you'll just learn to prepare them in a different way.

As I mentioned, I was a gourmet cook when I began to follow this Lifestyle. I fretted about what to do at parties, what to prepare for friends, how to eat at restaurants and what to do when I traveled. So, I converted my delicious gourmet recipes to fabulous raw dishes such as lasagna, pizzas, burgers, pies, crackers, cookies, pasta and other yummy creations. Some are quick and easy, requiring as few as five to 10 minutes to prepare; others are gourmet dishes and require a little more time. I believe that if we expect most people to eat raw and Living Foods over a long period of time, we have to make them taste good and we have to offer variety, especially during the transition period. I've really tried to make this Lifestyle fun, because people will be more inclined to stick with it.

The Living Foods Lifestyle encompasses a number of factors that help the body heal. Food is of the utmost importance, and certain foods are particularly good for people in a healing crisis. These foods are easy to digest and full of nourishment. They help detoxify and rebuild the body at the same time. You'll learn more about these healing foods later.

WHERE WILL I GET PROTEIN IF I DON'T EAT MEAT?

People obsess over protein. They worry they aren't getting enough when probably it's just the opposite – they're getting too much. I know it's confusing because "nutritional experts" give conflicting advice about how much protein humans should consume. With so much conflicting information out there, we must look inside ourselves for the truth, no matter what the so-called experts say.

Let's look for the truth. Many serious health problems such as cancer and heart disease are directly linked to eating too much meat. Meat is heavy and concentrated, requiring the greatest amount of time and energy to digest. Have you eaten a meal with meat and afterward felt you needed a nap? That's because meat requires so much energy to digest there's not enough left to keep your eyes open.

The body excretes less than an ounce of protein every 24 hours, so its actual requirements are low. If more protein is consumed than excreted, toxic waste builds up in the body. Harmful uric acid contributes to the body becoming more and more acidic. Bodies that are acidic are more likely to be diseased and unhealthy. The body needs all nutrients, not just protein.

Some people believe they must eat meat to be strong. How is it that elephants and oxen – some of the strongest and most powerful animals alive – eat only grasses and fruits? If they can build muscle and strength by eating a raw, vegetarian diet, why should humans be any different?

Humans need eight essential amino acids to build protein, not dead animal flesh. Vegetation is the original source of these amino acids. Most of the world's Oriental population lives on a meatless diet. The result is a significantly lower incidence of cancer and heart disease – and no evidence of any protein deficiency.

A majority of the eight essential amino acids are found in every fruit and vegetable. Some foods that contain all eight are: tomatoes, sweet potatoes, sunflower seeds, summer squash, sesame seeds, potatoes, peas, okra, nuts, kale, eggplant, corn, cauliflower, carrots, cabbage, brussels sprouts, bananas, and of course, wheatgrass. But vegetarianism does not guarantee good health when a person consumes a primarily cooked vegetarian diet. In fact, cooked vegetarian food can also be disease-forming. I know, because when I was diagnosed with cancer I was a vegan and weighed 192 pounds. Many vegetarians and vegans come to the Living Foods Institute in poor health, and are only able to restore their health when they stop cooking their food.

The human body needs carbohydrates for fuel, and meat provides virtually no carbohydrates. The body also requires fiber or cellulose for healthy colonic function, peristalsis and elimination. Meat has virtually no fiber. Humans require amino acids to build human protein. Meat provides complex animal protein, which must be broken down into its amino acid components by digestion. This is an inefficient use of the body's energy. By the way, the structure of amino acids is altered when meat is cooked, rendering them virtually useless, if not actually harmful.

Think about it: True carnivorous animals don't cook meat over the grill or in a frying pan. Carnivores have long, sharp claws and teeth for tearing and cutting animal flesh. Humans have hands and molars for picking fruit and chewing nuts. Carnivores have acid saliva to digest animal protein. Humans have alkaline saliva to digest starch. Carnivores have the ability to eliminate large quantities of uric acid, a by-product of protein digestion. Humans can eliminate only comparatively minute quantities of uric acid, which is highly toxic in the human body.

Would you still want to eat meat if you had to kill the animal yourself? I believe if that were the case we'd have a lot fewer meat eaters. If you're concerned about vitamin B-12, remember this: beneficial bacteria in a healthy colon will synthesize vitamin B-12.

You won't become protein deficient on the Living Foods Lifestyle. The sprouted nuts, seeds and berries as well as fruits and vegetables contain protein. Most people don't realize there's so much protein in plant life, and that it's easier to digest and assimilate than meat. The human digestive tract is not equipped to handle the digestion of meat properly. Most of the meat people eat actually rots and putrefies in the intestines, giving off large amounts of uric acid and other toxic by-products.

Most of the protein in sprouts and greens is in a pre-digested state. Because plant protein is in the form of simple amino acids, the body doesn't have to transform protein to amino acids. Also, plant protein is free from nucleo-proteins and does not form uric acid in the system. Excess uric acid can lead to gout, arthritis, rheumatism and other health problems. A low protein diet increases resistance to disease and helps build immunity to cancer.

It's interesting to me that one of the leading concerns among my students is the protein issue. They worry about not getting enough. The need for protein has been ingrained in us from the time we were taught about the four basic food groups. I call it the meat and protein propaganda. I believe meat producers have always been the ones pushing dead animal flesh on people. I think that instead of giving meat names such as hamburger and ribeye steaks, it should be labeled "dead ground cow flesh." I wonder how many people would still want to eat meat then?

You don't have to worry about not getting enough vitamins or protein when you eat high-energy, easy-to-digest blended Living Foods such as Energy Soup. Sprouted beans, avocados and greens have more than enough protein. Seed cheese is another good source of protein in the Living Foods Lifestyle. It's highly concentrated with protein and enzymes, so it's easy to digest. The body only absorbs about 20 to 30 percent of the protein in meat, but it absorbs 95 percent of nut and seed protein. In fact, it's possible to get too much protein in the Living Foods Lifestyle. For that reason, I recommend eating seed cheese sparingly.

Cooking meat can damage up to 85 percent of the protein,

which is sensitive to high temperatures. Living Foods protein is never cooked, so it's completely usable by the body and doesn't rot or putrefy in the intestines.

You might be surprised to know that seeds and beans have more protein than meat.

Following are the percentages of protein content in some popular foods:

Alfalfa Seeds	35% Protein
Mung Beans	27% Protein
Sunflower Seeds	27% Protein
Lentils	26% Protein
Split Peas	26% Protein
White Beans	24% Protein
Garbanzo Beans	24% Protein
Lean Beef	23% Protein
Fresh Fish	22% Protein
Chicken	21% Protein
Oats	18% Protein
Hard Wheat	14% Protein

It takes one acre of land to raise 40 pounds of animal flesh for human consumption. From the same acre you could raise 400 pounds of seeds, grains, nuts and beans. Why are we wasting so much land raising cattle just to kill and eat them? I'm sorry for every animal I ever ate before I became aware of what I was doing. When we eat animals that have been slaughtered we are eating their fear and anger, not just their flesh. Do you think this has anything to do with the anger and fear so many people feel today? Is this contributing to the violence among our youth? I'm glad I will never eat animals again.

LIVING FOODS AND THE PATH TO HEALING

When I adopted the Living Foods Lifestyle, I decided I would follow as closely as possible the guidelines that Ann Wigmore taught and practiced for more than 35 years. She worked with thousands of sick people and helped them heal. If it worked for her, I believed it would work for me. I wanted to heal quickly and was motivated in a way I had never been before. I was willing to do whatever it took, no matter how drastic it seemed. Changing from a mostly cooked diet to a completely raw and Living Foods diet was a drastic step for me. I found that having a positive attitude from the beginning helped me make the changes I needed to make. For the first six months I ate the four main healing foods every day. I believe these foods helped me heal the fastest. They are all simple, easy to prepare, basic foods.

- Energy Soup
- Rejuvelac
- Vege-Kraut
- Wheatgrass Juice

I also added green juices and watermelon juice to these four main foods. I believe that because I focused on eating these four main foods and adding these particular juices, I healed quickly. You may think eating just these foods sounds boring, but it's amazing how a serious disease can change your way of thinking. It was worth all my effort because it helped me heal quickly. It was, however, a tremendous challenge. I'm telling you this because you may feel the challenge is too great, or that it's too hard to make the changes. When you believe you will get a real benefit from making the changes, however, then no matter how difficult it may seem, it's worth it.

Don't think it was a breeze for me to eat these foods in the beginning. I didn't like any of them the first time I tasted them, and that's not uncommon. In fact, for a while I couldn't stand to look at them, smell them or be in the same room where they were being prepared. When I learned the four main foods and juices were my medicine, I kept eating them, even though I wasn't crazy about the taste. Actually, that's an understatement. I resorted to every trick in the book including holding my nose and gulping to get the food down. In other words, I did what I was told would work, not what was necessarily comfortable for me at that time. I stepped out of my comfort zone and it paid off. The more I ate these four main foods and drank these juices, the better I felt.

WHY ORGANIC?
OR, WHAT'S REALLY IN OUR FOOD?

The Living Foods Lifestyle isn't complicated or difficult. Following it will simplify your life, and save time and money. Your attitude will determine your success. If you look at it as a wonderful journey to health, you'll enjoy the process. If you look at it as a big pain, that's exactly what it will become. Choose a good attitude and you'll get great benefits.

Let's begin with the basics. First of all, eat only ORGANIC produce! Conventional produce can be genetically altered, filled with chemical fertilizers and sprayed with insecticides. Buying organic food is the only way to be sure you're getting real food without the toxins that can cause sickness and disease. If you can't pronounce a word on the label, or you don't know what it is, don't put it in your body. Long chemical names just sound scary. Get back to simplicity. Eating raw fruits and vegetables is easy. There's not much work in peeling a banana or slicing a tomato. Think of the energy bill reductions when you don't turn on the stove, oven, microwave, coffee maker, can opener or toaster oven.

I was in a popular chain grocery store a few months after I started the Living Foods Lifestyle. I saw a big box of nectarines that hadn't been unpacked and put out yet. On top of the box was a beautiful picture of a gorgeous, plump, juicy, inviting nectarine. At the bottom of the picture was fine print listing all the chemicals that had been sprayed on the fruit. I couldn't pronounce most of them, and had no idea what most were. But there were two names I did recognize – varnish and shellac. I don't know about you, but where I come from we use these products on furniture. They're certainly not something we'd consider eating. If we're going to eat varnish and shellac, why not just go to the hardware store and buy a pint or quart or gallon of each and turn it up and drink it? Ridiculous, isn't it? But we might as well drink it if we're going to eat fruit and vegetables that have been sprayed with it. It's the same with waxed fruit and vegetables. Growers tell you the wax is food grade and won't hurt you. I always ask this question, "Would you eat a candle?" No? Then why would you eat wax on vegetables and fruit? Peel any waxed fruit or vegetable.

In today's fast-paced world we turn to instant, frozen and prepared foods to feed our families and ourselves. We eat on the run and barely chew our food. Between the sugar and grease, we're pretty much drugged and clogged up by bad food. These foods may taste good, but they're making us sick. Many people know they should eat better, but they're addicted to bad foods and don't want to give them up. How sick do you have to get before you're willing to change what you eat?

Do you have any idea how dirty most restaurants are? I worked in the restaurant business for three years and let me tell you, it's filthy. I didn't work in greasy spoons either; I worked in the best restaurants. Do you think employees handling and preparing your food wash their hands after they visit the restroom? I don't think so. What if someone who handled your food had a serious, communicable disease? Would you know before it was too late?

When you prepare your own food, you know it's clean, and you know exactly what ingredients went into each recipe. You know if the food is fresh or spoiled. You know if the combinations of ingredients are good for you or not. When you eat food others have prepared, you have no idea what you're really eating. Take responsibility for preparing your food. If you're eating food someone else has prepared, be sure you know what's in it and the conditions under which it was prepared. If it says organic, check to be sure that it really is. Buy food from people you trust.

When I was eating all vegetables, I thought I was eating healthy. I wasn't. I still ate sweets and fats and processed food. Even if they said "organic" on the label, they were still void of any nutrition. I had to learn new things about food that I didn't know before, and I had to make changes in my food choices and the way I prepared my recipes. To sum it up, I had to develop a new relationship with food. I had to look at food as medicine and nourishment. I remind myself of that every time I put something in my mouth, and I'm going to remind you too.

Organic, raw and Living Foods are the best choice for health. It has worked for me, and thousands of others. The only way to see if it will work for you is to try it for yourself!

The Living Foods Lifestyle is more than a diet. I say this again and again because it's important for you to understand this is a Lifestyle. It's a total way of living that heals the body, the mind and the spirit. As important as food is for the body, it's equally important for the spirit and the mind. I mention this because I want you to understand that balance in all areas of life is important if you want to find real health and happiness. Just doing one thing, such as eating raw and Living Foods or drinking wheatgrass juice, isn't a magic key. Healing must involve the whole person – inside and out.

FOODS FOR THOSE IN A HEALING CRISIS

If you're not already sick, please don't wait until you are to make a change. I ignored my body and symptoms for years. I knew a lot of the things I did weren't good for me, but I did them anyway. Some things I thought were good for me, I found out weren't. I ate the Standard American Diet for years. Then I tried macrobiotics. I tried vegetarianism and veganism. I was always on a quest. Now that I know cooked food is dead – even cooked vegetables and fruits – and that dead food is devoid of most nutrition and all enzymes, I realize it was doing me no good.

For those in a healing crisis, or facing a serious disease, it's important to get serious about food choices. Raw foods are plentiful, and it's important to eat those particular foods the body needs for healing. The Living Foods Lifestyle for detoxification and rebuilding is based on a core group of four main foods and juices. These foods, when combined throughout the day, are nourishing, easy to digest, and offer a complete balance of vitamins, minerals, protein and fiber – everything a body needs to flourish.

Most people's digestive systems have virtually shut down or are operating at low capacity. Ann Wigmore recommends those in a health crisis should eat those four foods and drink juices. This gives the body time to rest and heal because it takes less energy to digest these foods. When combined, these particular foods provide complete nourishment. Later, as the body heals, other raw foods can be added gradually. In the beginning, simplicity is best to restore health. The body needs time to rest in order to heal, and not overtaxing your digestive system preserves energy for detoxing, healing and rebuilding. These foods are simple and easy to prepare. The recipes may be different from what you are used to, but once you get into the habit of eating these foods, they will become natural to you. I love saving time in the kitchen and growing the sprouts and greens myself.

E N E R G Y   S O U P

Energy Soup detoxifies and rebuilds the body. It's really a complete meal in a glass with vitamins, minerals and protein. Because it's blended, it's easy to digest. It's made from apple, sprouted mung beans, sprouted lentils, seaweed, dark green leafy vegetables, sunflower

sprouts, buckwheat lettuce sprouts, avocado and Rejuvelac or good filtered water. It nourishes the body completely, at the cellular level. It's
easy. It's simple. It's good for you. It would be a challenge to eat all
the ingredients that go into Energy Soup if they weren't blended
together. The greens alone would keep you busy chewing quite a
while. That's why I think Energy Soup is so great. I get all those
greens, and I don't have to worry if I'm chewing my food enough times
before I swallow. Most people, including me, have a bad habit of not
chewing food long enough. Digestion begins in the mouth and it's
important to chew food completely before you swallow. Chewing 50 to
100 times sounds drastic, doesn't it? But we need to chew each bite
until it becomes liquid in the mouth before swallowing. This is especially important for people with weak digestion.

When I was in my healing crisis during the first six months on
the Lifestyle, I tried to drink eight 8-ounce glasses of Energy Soup
every day. That's 64 ounces! In the beginning, I could barely get down
8 ounces, much less 64, but the more I ate Energy Soup, the better I
felt. After a few weeks, I was craving it. It really lives up to its name.
I can feel the energy after I drink it, and others tell me they can feel it
too. I've even had reports from some students who've seen sparks
jumping from the soup to their lips. That's some energy! Now that I'm
healed I don't drink as much Energy Soup each day as I used to, but I
try to drink one or two glasses. It makes me feel so good I can't resist it.
(See Energy Soup recipe on page 133.)

REJUVELAC

Rejuvelac is a fermented drink made with sprouted soft wheat
berries and good filtered water. It's one of the most important components of the Living Foods Lifestyle because it's a complete food, full of
protein, vitamins such as B, C and E, enzymes that help digest food,
minerals and friendly bacteria. We call Rejuvelac the "water" of the
Living Foods Lifestyle. While hydrating the body, it's also putting concentrated enzymes in our systems to help us digest food. The friendly
bacteria Rejuvelac puts into our bodies is essential for good colon
health. Instead of buying capsules, pills and powders from the store,
just make your own Rejuvelac. You'll get the good stuff you need with
every glass.

I drink Rejuvelac 15 to 20 minutes before eating, and my food digests easier. Because I clean my colon regularly, I drink Rejuvelac to replace the friendly bacteria. Doing this helped me get rid of Candida. I used to take acidophilus capsules to get good bacteria, but now I drink Rejuvelac. I try to drink eight 8-ounce glasses every day. Many times we think we are hungry when we really are just dehydrated. Not only can Rejuvelac rehydrate you, it can also provide great energy! It's more than just a drink; it's a complete food. If you're not drinking Rejuvelac each day, be sure to drink water. You won't get the nourishment from water that you do from Rejuvelac, but you will keep your body well hydrated. The more juicy fruits and vegetables you eat, the less water you need. But if you're eating a lot of cooked food, you will need a lot of water.

Blending Rejuvelac with fruits and vegetables prevents the loss of vitamins because Rejuvelac has a high vitamin E content and acts as an antioxidant. Rejuvelac's high enzyme level also helps tremendously with digestion.

(See Rejuvelac recipe on page 132.)

V E G E - K R A U T

I love this blend of fermented cabbage, juniper berries and seaweed, which I find soothing and easy to digest. Ann Wigmore created this recipe, which she called "Dr. Ann's Pink Sauerkraut." The pink color comes from mixing green and purple cabbage together. Vege-Kraut is full of digestive enzymes, pre-digested protein, lactic acid, vitamins, minerals and friendly bacteria. It builds bones and blood while helping restore balance in the intestinal tract. It, too, helped me overcome Candida. It's fermented, like Rejuvelac, and the friendly bacteria helps control yeast. Vege-Kraut also helped me get rid of parasites.

Fermented foods have been around for thousands of years and have helped many people around the world stay healthy. Now these foods are helping me. The colon requires Vege-Kraut to synthesize vitamins such as the Bs and produce valuable lactic acid. Though some doctors, teachers, books and diets are against fermented foods, I know they helped me, and I've seen them help so many others. I try to eat 8 ounces of Vege-Kraut throughout the day. Some days I want more; others I want less. I listen to my body and let it tell me what I need and how much of it. Trusting my inner voice to guide me is an important part of what the Living Foods Lifestyle has taught me. I am much more relaxed now and not worried if I'm getting enough of this or that. My body tells me what it needs and I give it what it asks for. As a result, my energy is high, my skin looks great, and my eyes are bright. I feel fabulous!

(See Vege-Kraut recipe on page 135.)

WHEATGRASS JUICE

Wheatgrass Juice is liquid chlorophyll that's full of vitamins and minerals in the purest, easiest-to-digest form there is. I believe it's much better to get vitamins and minerals in a fresh, alive form rather than from a pill, powder or potion. I used to take double handfuls of vitamin pills every day until I began practicing the Living Foods Lifestyle. Now I get all my vitamins from wheatgrass juice and Living Foods. To get the juice out of the blades, put them through a juicing machine specially designed to extract the juice from wheatgrass. You can't use an ordinary juicer to juice wheatgrass, but the Omega Juicer will juice fruits, vegetables and wheatgrass. There are also machines that juice only wheatgrass.

Wheatgrass juice, along with Living Foods, has helped me restore my body to perfect health. I drink 1 to 2 ounces each day, and I also implant 2 to 4 ounces into my colon each day. During the first six months, I drank 2 to 4 ounces and implanted 8 to 16 ounces daily. Implanting wheatgrass directly into the colon after cleansing with an enema is one of the most potent ways to benefit from its properties. I believe this is the best way to get the full benefit of wheatgrass juice. It cleanses the colon walls, pulls out toxins and nourishes all at the same time. This is especially important for people who can't keep anything on their stomach because of nausea.

I've tried taking wheatgrass juice orally and rectally and compared the detoxing effects. I did much more intense detoxing when I implanted it into my colon. Also, because I wanted to get 4 to 8 ounces or more of wheatgrass in my body each day, it was easier to implant it than to drink it. **It's important to cleanse the colon with an enema or colonic before implanting wheatgrass juice.** Implant the wheatgrass within 30 minutes of cleansing the colon and hold it for 10 to 15 minutes. Some, or all, of it may stay in the colon. The rest may be eliminated. The body will keep what it needs. I also do vaginal implants each day with 1 to 2 ounces of wheatgrass, which helps eliminate fibroids and tumors.

Don't think wheatgrass juice is a miracle by itself. It must be combined with raw and Living Foods to provide real, healing effects. People who think they can eat as they please and make up for it by drinking wheatgrass juice are fooling themselves. It takes more than just one thing to heal the body. Everything must work together in harmony.

Wheatgrass juice contains more than 100 elements and vitamins such as A, B-complex, C, E and K and minerals such as sodium, calcium, iron, magnesium, phosphorus, sulphur, cobalt and zinc. It's rich in protein, and contains all 17 essential amino acids (eight of which our bodies can synthesize from the food we eat). Enzymes and amino acids are responsible for cell renewal, creating hormones, and building muscles, blood and organs. **Wheatgrass juice is similar to human blood. One of the only differences is that blood contains iron as its nucleus and wheatgrass juice contains magnesium.**

Drink wheatgrass juice on an empty stomach and wait 15 to 20 minutes before eating. People who are allergic to wheat shouldn't have problems with wheatgrass because gluten and other elements present in the grain aren't present in the wheatgrass.

Wheatgrass cleanses, rebuilds and neutralizes toxins. It can dissolve scars in the lungs and help reduce high blood pressure. It's a purifier and detergent on and in the body. It helps overcome dandruff and prevents tooth decay. It helps relieve sore throats, and disinfects and cleans out bacteria and viruses. It helps clean the bloodstream and aids in digestion. It can be used as a mouthwash, and it freshens the breath. It's wonderful for cleansing and beautifying the skin, and can help overcome aging. Wheatgrass juice can help remove toxic metals such as lead, cadmium, mercury, aluminum and copper that have been stored in the body. It helps build white blood cells when combined with raw and Living Foods.

I can't say enough good things about wheatgrass. It's easy to grow at home, indoors, and it's economical when you grow it yourself. Pets love it too, and it's good for them. Wheatgrass is a wonderful medicine for the body.

Wheatgrass is abundant in vitamins, minerals, trace elements and enzymes. It is easy to digest and a high quality medicine for the body. Again, wheatgrass is rich in protein and contains all 17 amino acids. The human body synthesizes eight of these essential amino acids. Enzymes and amino acids are responsible for renewing cells, creating hormones and building muscles, blood and human organs. The amino acids used by the human body are:

- **Isoleucine:** Helps produce other amino acids, aids mental health, balances protein in adults, and is essential for growth in infants.
- **Leucine:** Helps maintain high energy, keeps you alert and awake.
- **Lysine:** For immune system response and anti-aging qualities.
- **Phenylalanine:** Helps the thyroid gland produce thyroxin, a hormone good for mental balance and emotional calm.
- **Theronine:** Stimulates smooth digestion and assimilation of food and metabolism.
- **Tryptophane:** Stimulates digestion, works with B vitamins to help calm nerves, builds rich blood, healthy skin and hair.
- **Valine:** Protects against nervousness, mental fatigue, emotional outbursts and insomnia. Activates the brain and helps with muscle coordination.
- **Methionine:** Helps hair grow, promotes mental calmness, helps cleanse and regenerate the liver and kidneys.

The other nine amino acids also found in wheatgrass are:
- **Alanine:** A blood builder.
- **Arginine:** Vital for men; found in seminal fluids.
- **Aspartic Acid:** Helps convert food into energy.
- **Glutamic Acid:** Provides for smooth metabolic function and improves mental balance.
- **Glycine:** Helps cells convert oxygen into energy.
- **Histidine:** Affects hearing and nervous functions.
- **Proline:** Becomes glutamic acid and performs the same benefits.
- **Serine:** Stimulates the brain and nervous functions.
- **Tyrosine:** Helps form hair and skin. Prevents cellular aging.

Wheatgrass contains a full spectrum of vitamins and minerals and is not toxic in any amount.

Wheatgrass creates an unfavorable environment for bacteria to grow, making it an effective healer. In 1962 Ann Wigmore started growing wheatgrass indoors. More than 30 years ago, scientists working independently in Germany, South Africa and Australia drafted reports showing that all the nutrients necessary for normal human body function could be found in grasses and weeds of various kinds. That meant no more need for artificial vitamins. Wheatgrass contains all 103 elements known to man. For more information about wheatgrass, I recommend *The Wheatgrass Book*, by Ann Wigmore. In it you'll learn how Wigmore discovered the properties of wheatgrass and used that knowledge to help thousands of people.

WHEATGRASS AND THE DETOXIFICATION PROCESS

Don't be alarmed if you experience detoxification symptoms when you begin using wheatgrass and Living Foods. It's normal to feel some discomfort during detox and symptoms can vary from person to person. Some symptoms I had were headaches, nausea, diarrhea, low energy, rash, pimples, itching, ringing in my ears, sore throat, chills, fever, mucous and sleeplessness. I found enemas and colonics helped detox symptoms pass quickly. I did my heavy-duty detoxing in about the first seven days. After that I continued to detox, but I didn't have the same severe symptoms. Whatever you do, don't stop the detox process because you think you're allergic to wheatgrass or Living Foods. These symptoms are coming from toxins being released into your system. Sometimes people want to give up when detox starts, but sooner or later, they have to go through it. Toxins that aren't released will continue to make you sick.

GROWING WHEATGRASS IN YOUR KITCHEN

Soak about 2 cups of organic hard winter wheat berries in good filtered water for 8 to 12 hours. (Note: hard winter wheat is used to grow wheatgrass and soft wheat is used to make Rejuvelac.) Soak in glass or stainless steel pots (no plastic or aluminum) and cover the container's opening with mesh, cheesecloth or net. This will help you fill the container and pour off water without losing the berries. Cover the berries with double the amount of water as berries, to give them room to expand. Soak for 8 to 12 hours then pour off the water and rinse well. Turn the container to a 45-degree angle so the rest of the water continues to drain. Don't let the berries completely cover the mouth of the container when you turn it on its side. This allows air cir-culation, which is important in the sprouting process. Rinse the berries twice each day, morning and afternoon, and continue sprout-ing until the tail is about the same length as the berry. When the berries have sprouted, they are ready to plant.

Place an inch or so of organic soil in a planting tray with good drainage. Sprinkle with about a tablespoon of dulse flakes or granu-lated kelp. Minerals from the seaweed are good for the wheatgrass. Put another inch of soil on top of that and pat down. Spread sprout-ed seeds evenly atop the soil. Don't pile seeds on top of one another, but do cover all the soil well with seeds. Water well with good water. (Don't use unfiltered tap water. The water you use on your wheatgrass will be the same water you will consume in the liquid wheatgrass.) Don't water the wheatgrass again until the third day. Cover the plant-ing tray with another tray or a piece of cardboard to keep all light out for three days. You can also use wet newspaper, but only use the black and white pages, not color. I prefer to cover the trays with another tray so I don't have to worry about toxicity in the chemicals used to print newspaper. Let the tray sit for three days. On the third day remove the top tray so the grass can get light. When you remove the top, water well, being careful not to over-water. Drain well, and set the tray in an area that receives good light. Direct sunlight isn't necessary. When you first remove the top, the wheatgrass will have grown about 2 inches and will be yellow. When the tray begins to get light, the blades will quickly turn green. Leave the top off and continue watering each day until the wheatgrass is about 6 to 7 inches high. Then it's ready to cut.

Use a serrated edge knife and cut right above the berries. Store in the refrigerator in plastic bags with air holes punched in them. The wheatgrass will stay fresh for about seven days. If it begins to turn yel-low, discard it because it's breaking down. Check the temperature of your refrigerator to be sure it's cold enough. This will keep your grass fresher for a longer period of time. Juice wheatgrass immediately before use; it's best within 15 to 20 minutes of juicing. In warm, humid climates mold can sometimes be a problem when growing wheatgrass. Try using a fan to keep air circulating around the wheatgrass. This will help cut down on or eliminate mold completely. If some mold does grow on the wheatgrass, it will be close to the bottom of the blade, just above the seeds. Cut above the mold when harvesting the wheatgrass, and it should be fine.

G R E E N   J U I C E S ,   W A T E R M E L O N   J U I C E   A N D   T H E   F O U R   M A I N   F O O D S

The juices of dark, green, leafy vegetables are cleansing and nourishing to the body. Aside from Rejuvelac, green juices are my favorite beverages. They're refreshing and energizing, and I feel clean when I drink them. I like to take one to two days each week and drink just green juices all day. This type of "fasting" on green juice is good for the body. It allows the digestive system to rest as it nourishes, detoxifies and rebuilds the body. Plus, it's easy on the system. I recommend you invest in a good juicer, and juice organic, fresh, alive juices each day. Drink your juice as soon as you juice it for the maximum nutrition and benefits.

One of my favorite juice combinations is kale, cucumber, celery and parsley. Green juices will detox the body quickly, so go slowly. For the first two months on the Living Foods Lifestyle I ate mostly Energy Soup and Vege-Kraut and drank Rejuvelac and Wheatgrass Juice. I waited until after I'd done significant detoxing to incorporate green juices. Too many green juices early on would've made my detoxing go too fast, something Ann Wigmore warns against. In the beginning of her work, she recommended green juice fasting. Then she found most people were so toxic and deficient that fasting was too drastic. That's when she began recommending blended Energy Soup. Detoxing still happens, but at a slower pace. Listen to your own body and decide what's best for you.

Watermelon is classified as both a fruit and vegetable and it's the most alkaline of all. It's especially effective in helping overcome acidic conditions in the body. Watermelon is also a wonderful resource for natural water. The rind is rich in protein, enzymes, minerals, chlorophyll and vitamins A, B and C. It's easy to digest, even for people with poor digestion. It's wonderful for the kidneys, bladder and urinary tract, helping to eliminate harmful uric acid. Juice the entire melon, including the rind. Fasting on watermelon juice for one or two days or more is beneficial to your body. Because I had Candida and didn't need to eat a lot of sugary fruits, I diluted the watermelon juice with half Rejuvelac or water.

The four main healing foods, green juices and watermelon juice will detox and rebuild the body quickly. Again, this is what I suggest for anyone in a healing crisis. It sounds drastic – and it is – but it takes measures such as this to heal a sick body. As you begin adding other raw and Living Foods to your diet, you may notice changes in your level of detoxing and in your energy levels. After six months of mostly the four main foods, I began adding other foods to my diet. I found that some foods, even though they were raw, soaked, sprouted, etc., were too rich for my body. I ate soaked nuts until I noticed I developed mucous after eating them. When I cut out the nuts, the mucous stopped. I believe the nuts were too acidic for my body. I feel better not eating nuts, and even though I used to love them, I have no desire for them now. Ann Wigmore warns about nuts being too acidic and concentrated for cancer patients. I'm listening to my body and paying attention to the signals it sends. Now I know when something is good for me, and when it's not. Listen to your body and your inner voice. You have all the answers inside.

CHOICES FOR THOSE NOT IN A HEALING CRISIS

If you aren't in a healing crisis, then, in addition to the four main foods, green juices and watermelon juices, you can eat as much raw and Living Foods as you like. If you're facing a healing crisis, the more green foods you eat, the better. Salads and tasty raw dishes will add variety and flavor to your meals. The recipes at the end of this book will give you an example of some delicious favorites of my students. I created these recipes to help people who are transitioning off cooked food. They are gourmet, tasty and satisfying. I don't eat these recipes myself. I used to, but as my body has changed I've lost my taste and desire for rich foods. I eat simply now, and I enjoy just having a fruit or vegetable by itself. Use these foods when you're giving up cooked food and they will help you make the transition.

My advice is to keep it simple. Make it easy on your digestive system by eating only one or two foods at the same time. Mixing several different foods in one sitting can be hard on the body. Less is best. The more different types of foods you put into the body at one time, the harder they will be to digest. I know it's important for most people to have variety in their food, and for them to get excited about raw and Living Foods, these dishes must taste good and look good. That's why I created delicious recipes to help beat boredom. As you experiment with these recipes, pay attention to how you feel after eating them. Now when I eat too many types of foods at once, or too many concentrated foods, I have gas and I'm tired. Even Living Foods and raw foods can be hard on the body when not properly combined.

Listen to your body when you eat. Pay attention to how you feel afterward. Is your energy high, or are you tired? Do you have gas, bloating or indigestion? Do you sleep well, or are you restless? Do you wake up refreshed, or still exhausted? When you eat well, do you feel good? When you eat poorly, do you feel bad? It isn't that complicated. Learn to listen to your inner voice. How much is feeling good worth to you? What price are you willing to pay for good health? Each of us is unique and our bodies respond to different foods in different ways. What works for one person may not work for another. Go slowly, experiment with different foods, and see how you feel.

When adding additional foods to your diet, opt simply for green, leafy vegetables. Keep sweet fruits to a minimum and avoid them altogether for a while if you have Candida or cancer. How long you must stay away from fruits will differ for each person. I didn't eat fruit for four to six months. When I was tested again, the Candida was gone. Gradually I began adding fruit back into my diet and now I eat fruit whenever I want it. I'm just careful not to overdo it.

Concentrated foods such as nuts and seeds can be fatty and hard on the digestive system, so use good judgment when eating them. I found nuts and seeds difficult to digest. Although I like the way they taste, I don't like the way I feel after I eat them, so I stay away from them as much as possible. There may come a time when my body can better tolerate concentrated foods, but in the meantime I plan to keep it simple.

A BODY-MIND-SPIRIT
CONNECTION

ALL ABOUT THE COLON

I believe, as Ann Wigmore did, that all diseases originate in the colon. Actually, I believe they begin in the mind, with toxic and negative thoughts and emotions, and then progress to the colon. Think about the diet most people consume – highly processed, refined, deficient in fiber, treated with chemicals, irradiated, genetically altered with no enzymes – and you'll see the colon has absolutely no chance of functioning properly. If your colon isn't working, your body is filling with toxic waste and becoming deprived of nourishment. It may be sluggish, sick and diseased.

I'll bet only a very small percentage of the population has healthy colons. If most other colons are like mine was, there are a lot of toxic waste dumps out there, loaded with impacted, putrefy-ing, decaying, toxic material, toxic gas, parasites, yeast, bacteria and other unhealthy substances.

It's not a pleasant thought, is it? Well, it's the truth.

Fecal material can become hard and impacted if the colon doesn't eliminate regularly and efficiently. When this happens impurities can be absorbed into the bloodstream. When blood becomes polluted with junk from a diseased colon it can spread throughout the body, which can make you sick.

HEALTHY COLON, HEALTHY LIFE

After struggling to adjust to Living Foods, a miracle occurred. I realized I actually came to like these foods – I even craved them. After working to change my eating habits for the first few weeks, I became more and more accustomed to these wonderful new foods.

My body responded quickly. For the first time in years I began to feel what it was like to be nourished at the cellular level and to feel really good. I began to look younger; my wrinkles softened and some even disappeared. My tumors were shrinking, and the age or liver spots on my hands and arms were fading. I discovered the reason I got these spots in the first place was because of my dirty, toxic colon. That sounds charming, doesn't it? Just think: If the toxic waste in the colon can't be eliminated in the normal way, it seeps out through the skin. Yuck!

Colon cleansing is not something most people like to talk about, much less do, but it is important to healing. Over time it's something I've become quite comfortable with. Is your colon clean or dirty? It's dirty if you haven't been cleaning it regularly and eating the right foods. "Oh no," you may be thinking, "She's not going to talk about enemas and stuff like that, is she?" Yes, yes I am! So keep that mind open and let's address another reason we get sick. Let's talk about the dirty, toxic waste dump we call our colon.

Did you know that almost everyone, even thin people, has between 5 to 30 pounds of impacted fecal matter in their colon? Extremely obese people may have 50, 60, 70 or more pounds of toxic matter seeping back through colon walls, backing up to the liver, dirtying the blood and making them sick. Think this sounds disgusting? Just think what toxic waste can do to your body if you don't get rid of it.

When I first heard about the Living Foods Lifestyle, I could understand why it was important to eat Living Food, but I didn't think much about my colon or how it related to my health. Now I truly understand why we must remove toxic, impacted fecal waste if we want to get healthy. Eating organic, raw and Living Foods alone is not enough to heal the body. Cleansing the colon is just as important as eating the right foods.

When I was a little girl I remember my mother giving me Milk of Magnesia for constipation. I hated that stuff. I would kick and scream to keep from taking it, but it didn't help. She made me take it anyway. Sometimes I would throw up as soon as I swallowed it. I would always gag. Those are unpleasant memories, but I realize my mother was doing what she thought was best for me. I have a wonderful mother who always had the best intentions, just as I always have the best intentions for my son. But now I realize a lot of things that seemed right at the time, weren't. My mother knew it was important for me to have regular bowel movements. If I didn't, Milk of Magnesia was her remedy. I vaguely remember getting enemas when I was little. While I don't have any negative memories about them, the thought of that Milk of Magnesia still makes me cringe.

I've found through working with many different types of people that most of us have an aversion to talking about the colon, enemas and colonics. We're embarrassed or ashamed of the inside of our bodies and anything that has to do with bowel movements. This is something I hope to help people become more comfortable with. That's why I always include an informative, "entertaining" class during my 10-Day Training on enemas and colonics. When I do this class, we laugh, joke and have fun talking about enemas. My husband, bless his heart, has given the enema a new name. He calls it the "fanny flush." Call it enema, fanny flush or anything you like, just do it!

It's time we become more comfortable with cleansing our bodies from the inside out. Getting professional colonics and doing personal enemas at home is an important part of healing. Would you go all your life without bathing or brushing your teeth? Of course not, so why go all your life without cleaning the inside of your body? The inside is even more important than the outside. When the body is dirty and toxic inside, it manifests in symptoms and diseases. The cleaner you keep the inside of your body and the better you nourish your body, the better it will run, and the better you'll feel. I believe I could never have experienced total health without systematic colon cleansing. Getting rid of the bad stuff you've accumulated over the years is just as important as putting in the good stuff – raw, Living, organic fresh fruit and vegetables.

The colon is an important part of the digestive system and the major organ for elimination. It absorbs nutrients, eliminates wastes, creates valuable products such as vitamins, keeps unfriendly bacteria in check and performs many other complex functions that regulate the entire body's health. Poor health can result if any of these functions does not occur properly. A wonderful book I recommend all my students read is *Colon Health* by Dr. Norman Walker. Please take the time to learn how to take care of your colon – the rewards will be great.

FROM CRITTERS TO CONSTIPATION:
SYMPTOMS OF AN UNHEALTHY COLON

Parasites can also be a persistent problem. These little creatures really come alive when the colon is impacted with decaying material. They can embed themselves in waste matter and in the outer layers of the colon wall. It can take great effort and time to get rid of them. If you're tired all the time, you may be infested with parasites. They can drain your energy by interfering with nutrient absorption.

If you want to get rid of parasites you have to get rid of decay and deprive parasites of anything to feed on. Did you know parasites and worms can range from specks to a few feet long? Sounds disgusting, doesn't it? That's what I thought, too, especially when I found out I was infested with these critters. I got rid of parasites by eating foods such as garlic, ginger and cayenne pepper with my raw and Living Foods. Remember, if you don't have decaying, putrefied matter in your colon, parasites won't have anything to eat. You may think you don't have parasites, but don't be too sure. Most people do. Get tested for parasites and Candida or other diseases through bioenergetic assessments or blood cell analysis. Find out what's really going on inside your body. Once you know, you can take measures to correct the problems.

Gas isn't a topic anyone likes to discuss, but it's a problem many of us are plagued with. Improperly digested food decays, producing gas and toxic chemical reactions. Toxic gases can be absorbed into the bloodstream, creating a toxic condition for the entire body. Gas can cause a bloated, uncomfortable feeling. What do you do in public? It can be embarrassing when you need to pass gas.

Speaking of gas, how does yours smell? A foul, rotten smell is directly related to the foods you're eating. Meat eaters have incredibly bad smelling gas. I used to have a big problem with gas before I began eating Living Foods. Even for the first month or so I had terrible gas on and off when I ate the healing foods. What I discovered was that as the good foods stirred up impacted fecal matter in my colon, it created gas. Every time I got gas I'd remember to take an enema. That helped get rid of the gas and more of the impacted waste. The cleaner I got my colon, the less gas I had. Today I rarely have gas unless I combine foods poorly – something that happens from time to time. Usually it's the fancy recipes that give me gas. Simple foods always digest with ease. Even if I do get gas now, it has no smell. My colon is clean and my health reflects it. Always remember to drink plenty of Rejuvelac and eat lots of Vege-Kraut to put friendly bacteria back in your colon. When you clean the colon, you wash out good and bad bacteria alike.

Proper food combining is also an effective way to help control gas. Eating starches with proteins or fruits is not good food combining and can cause gas and digestion problems. For optimum digestion, eat every food alone. Your body is set up to handle just one food at a time. Eat fruits independently from vegetables. Eat melons separately from any other food. Leafy greens combine well with just about every other vegetable and are an aid to digestion. The best thing to do is listen to your own body. If you get gas and bloating after eating certain foods, you know that's not a good combination for you.

With raw and Living Foods you can ease up on some food combining laws because the food is not cooked. One example would be putting fruit in Energy Soup. This seems to blend and digest well, even though it isn't ideal food combining.

Constipation is a big problem for many people. I never thought I had a problem with constipation because I had a bowel movement every day. Just like babies, however, we should have bowel movements every time we eat – at least three or four a day. Even though I was having a bowel movement every day, I was still impacted and constipated.

Most people think having a bowel movement once a day is OK, but it's not! Waste must be eliminated from the body before it can putrefy and create conditions that allow "unfriendly" bacteria such as yeast, parasites and gas to take over. Food becomes compact and difficult to eliminate the longer it stays in the body. Laxatives aren't the answer because they don't get rid of constipation. They're just another false "quick fix" that does more to aggravate the body than help it. In fact, laxatives are poisons to the body and the only reason you have a bowel movement when you take a laxative is that the body recognizes it as a toxin and tries to get it out as fast as possible. A good, Living Foods diet has been my answer for good elimination.

If you want to restore your colon to perfect health, eat Living Foods, get regular colonics and do enemas and wheatgrass implants!

YOU WANT ME TO PUT WHAT WHERE?!

When I first heard about colonics and enemas I was repulsed. I didn't want to think about, talk about or do anything about cleaning out my colon. But the more I learned, the more I realized that if I didn't clean out my colon, all the good, organic, nutritious, raw and Living Food wouldn't do me any good. I had to clean out the toxic waste dump – my colon – in order to restore my health.

My first colonic wasn't the horror I imagined. It was gentle and dignified. My colonic therapist was caring and knowledgeable. She helped me relax and let go of the old waste matter that had been making me sick. After a few colonics, I started feeling better. It actually took about four colonics before I really began to release the stuff that had been in my colon for years. In addition to getting rid of impacted fecal waste, I also detoxed emotional baggage I had been carrying around for years.

I found massage therapy with castor oil on my abdomen was effective in helping me release during the colonic. I received a massage from a massage therapist who knew how to help the body release hardened, impacted waste. Because I didn't release much of anything during my first three colonics, my colon therapist recommended I get a massage before my next session. I did and wow! I released 45 minutes worth of stuff that ranged from brown to solid, jet black.

The black substance was old, impacted matter that had been in there for years. If I hadn't seen it with my own eyes, I wouldn't believe it. I had read other's stories about releasing gross stuff from the colon, but I had to experience it myself to truly believe. I now always use the essential oil blends, Ab-Ez and Let It Go, that I have had developed to help the colon to relax and let go of the waste. These blends also help us to let go of buried emotions that can be making us sick.

Did you know we store emotions in our colons? As we clean the colon, we clean up other areas of life. I was holding all kinds of bad feelings in my colon, including anger and resentment from a bad divorce. As I cleaned my colon, these feelings came rushing out. I was finally able to let them go and heal this longstanding unhappiness and resentment. When I began giving myself enemas and wheatgrass implants (juicing wheatgrass and implanting it directly into the colon) every day, my health began to improve dramatically. Wheatgrass is a powerful medicine, and its vitamins and minerals can help clean the colon as it nourishes the body.

Many people question giving themselves an enema, but I wouldn't think about going a day without cleansing my colon. In the beginning I was so impacted that I hardly had a bowel movement unless I did an enema. After a couple of months my colon got stronger, and regular bowel movements returned. It amazes me that even after a good bowel movement there is still so much fecal waste left in the colon. That's why I always do an enema, even after a bowel movement, so I can get all the waste material out. I believe this is one key to optimum health.

If you've heard enemas and colonics will keep you from having regular bowel movements, stop worrying – it isn't true. In fact, colonics and enemas actually strengthened my colon. I believe we should be more concerned with leaving toxic waste in the colon than with the process of removing it. It's amazing that so much waste is in our bodies. One of my students told our class that the great actress, Mae West, was asked how she maintained such beautiful skin. She said, "I do an enema every day!" People thought she was kidding or crazy, but Mae West did something for her health it would do all of us a lot of good to do every day. Do enemas – be healthy and beautiful!

After three or four colonics I began to release old, impacted waste. As I said, it was almost solid black. The colon therapist said the black sludge had been there the longest. At one session I released solid black gunk for at least 15 minutes. It blew me away. After that session I felt so light, I thought I could float on air.

If you're turned off by colonics and wheatgrass implants, think of all the diseases that begin in a dirty colon, including colon cancer. I don't know anyone who wants to experience that devastating disease. Maybe thinking about the consequences of disease will encourage you to do things that will keep you healthy, even if it's something different, such as a colonic or enema.

You've heard me say it before, and I'll say it again, step out of your comfort zone and make changes that will restore your health. I talk to people about making lifestyle changes by eating better, thinking better and cleaning out their colons. Some of them tell me they would get serious about making changes if they had a serious disease. Why wait until you're really sick? Prevention is the best route to take. If we all took more responsibility for our health before we got sick, we could avoid a lot of pain, suffering, misery and expense. Don't wait until it's too late. Take care of yourself now!

GET A NEW BODY – GET A NEW LIFE

DESIRABLE BODY WEIGHT IS ATTAINABLE

I used to be a yo-yo dieter. I'd lose a pound and gain back two. I'll bet I've lost and gained at least one or two people in my lifetime. It was one endless, depressing struggle after another. I wish I'd known about the Living Foods Lifestyle when I was a teenager. I could've saved myself a lot of grief about my weight. Of course there's always the issue of whether I would have followed the Living Foods Lifestyle even if I'd known about it then. I think it took something life-threatening to get my attention.

As you already know, what attracted me to the Living Foods Lifestyle was not my weight problem. Even though I knew I needed to lose weight, I had no motivation to do it. What did get my attention was the breast and cervical tumors. I wanted to get rid of those as quickly as possible. The wonderful surprise was that when I ate raw and Living Foods, I lost weight. In just two weeks I lost 23 pounds and I continued to lose another 52 pounds over the next 60 days.

That sounds like a lot of weight loss in a short amount of time, doesn't it? I've always heard it's not healthy to lose weight so fast, and that quick weight loss comes back almost as quickly as it went away. That was true when I was doing all those crazy diets, but with Living Foods the weight has stayed off and I've become stronger, firmer and

JUNE 2009 SPECIAL CONVOCATION
ADDENDUM

ROY
THOMSON
HALL
Toronto, Ontario

Thursday,
June 18, 2009
2:00 p.m.

The following candidate will be present to receive their call during this ceremony:

Sherif Ragai Ashamalla
Jordan Avrum Druxerman
Jeffrey Philip Viater

The following candidate will not be present to receive his call during this ceremony:

Dov Asher Fried

incredibly energized. One reason I shed so much weight was because I did colonics and enemas. I probably had 20 pounds of impacted matter in my colon.

I learned another good lesson through this – enzymes are key to losing or gaining weight. When I began to eat raw and Living Foods, full of enzymes and complete nutrition, the pounds just melted away. Maybe the fact that I stopped eating candy bars and potato chips and drinking martinis had a little to do with it too!

LIVING FOODS CAN HELP YOU GAIN WEIGHT

Did you know there are actually people trying to gain weight? For each of us who has battled with losing weight, there's another who'd do almost anything to gain weight. I've worked with people who have been thin all their lives, and also with those challenged by weight loss from AIDS, cancer or other serious diseases. These people also have hope. I've seen many people gain weight back on the Living Foods Lifestyle. Enzymes are the key to weight gain and weight loss. Many people who have had problems with weight loss or weight gain on every other program have experienced tremendous success with this Lifestyle.

It's important to customize food choices and practice good food combining to achieve your goals. Some foods will help you lose weight and some will help you gain. No matter where you are with your weight, whether you need to lose, gain or maintain, I believe the Living Foods Lifestyle can help you do it with ease. By developing a new understanding of and relationship with food, I've accomplished one of my greatest goals: to become fit and healthy. You can too!

GIVE ME STRENGTH – AND FLEXIBILITY!

Fitness trainers, body builders and exercise enthusiasts ask how this lifestyle can help them gain muscle mass, especially if they eat no meat. "Where will I get protein?" they wonder. Think about this: Some of the largest, most powerful animals in the world – gorillas and elephants – eat only raw, green vegetation. They don't eat meat or cooked food, yet they build thousands of pounds of solid muscle. A wonderful book, *Raw Power*, by Steve Arlin, explores this subject in detail. I recommend it to anyone concerned with building muscle while eating raw and Living Foods. I've found that as I've lost weight I've increased my muscle mass, my skin continues to tone up and my body gets better and better.

For a while I worked with free weights and weight machines. I did aerobics, and I even worked out with a trainer. Now, instead of pumping iron, I practice Bikram Yoga. I had read about the benefits of yoga but had never tried it until February 2001 (my 2001 New Year's resolution was to take up yoga). Yoga has allowed me to firm and tone my body while building incredible flexibility, strength, endurance, focus and concentration. Each posture works on different internal organs, and I feel that as I'm exercising I'm continuing to heal my body, mind and spirit.

In Bikram Yoga, the room is heated so while I'm doing the postures, I sweat a lot. I never sweated that much when I worked out in the gym. Even when I did aerobics I would only sweat a little. With Bikram Yoga, my body pours sweat, and I feel I am detoxing with every move. I needed to work on flexibility and not just building muscle. My flexibility has improved and every day I can feel parts of my body stretch that have never stretched before.

When I practice yoga each day, I feel the benefits in my life. Even on the days I miss class, I'm still able to reach and bend with ease. Yoga is the perfect exercise for me. I'm addicted now, and it's wonderful to have an addiction that's so good for me. I urge you to explore exercise and get your body moving.

THE BODY-MIND-SPIRIT CONNECTION – WHAT DOES IT MEAN?

So much pain and misery could be avoided if we paid more attention to what we put in our mouths and what we let come out of our mouths – our words. What we eat does make a difference in how we feel and look. What we eat does make a difference in our health. What we eat is either keeping us healthy or killing us. What we say and think also impacts our health. To have health we must expect it, think it and live it. What we let get into our minds is just as important as what we put into our mouths, maybe more so.

We are bombarded with television, radio and printed media that promote drugs and bad food. We look at and listen to these commercials and we buy these products. Watch enough TV and you might just start believing that Coke is the "real thing," or that a milk mustache is cool. Be careful about what you let into your mind. Be careful about what you believe.

What we put into our mouth is important for good health. Just as important are our thoughts and words. In a way, what comes out of our mouths is actually more important than what goes in them because what we think and say is directly connected to our health. Many times people will come to the Living Foods Institute 10-Day Program thinking they're only going to learn new ways to prepare food and that hope alone will make them well.

They come to understand that disease begins in the mind. Eating organic, raw and Living Foods will not heal the body if the mind is full of toxic thoughts. One of the first steps in healing is not only to forgive others, but ourselves as well. Toxic thoughts of jealousy, anger, resentment, hostility and unhappiness are just as bad for us as eating meat, dairy and sugar. You can eat the right foods all day long, but if you're harboring anger against others, you won't get well.

Emotional detoxification is an important part of healing. Some people carry thoughts in their heads that are making them sick. These toxic thoughts are eating away at them and preventing them from living a happy, fulfilled life. When you are ready to heal, you must start with your mind.

Thoughts are things; every thought and word you speak manifests into your life. Positive thoughts produce positive results. Negative thoughts produce negative results. Having faith and believing that this Lifestyle works is crucial to its success. Fear and doubt will hold you back. Knowing that you are healed, recognizing that there is a greater power in the universe – God – and that this power is working in you, around you and through you for healing, is one of the most important steps. **Believe that it works and it does.**

Daily spiritual work in the form of prayer, meditation, affirmations and visualizations to confirm your health is important. First, know you are in a total and perfect state of health. Take the time each day to do this spiritual work – it's far more significant than what you eat. It's the single most important thing you can do for yourself and your life. What you feed your mind – your thoughts and words – creates health or disease. You hold the key to the power of healing within your mind. Learn to use this to create exactly the life and health you want.

KNOWING IS MORE POWERFUL THAN BELIEVING

Believing in something is wonderful, but it's not enough to just believe. When you go beyond just believing to knowing that something is true, when you "feel" it in every bone in your body, in every cell, then and only then will you create what you want. The power is in the "knowing." Stay focused on what you really want. Write down in positive affirmations what you want to create, i.e. "I know I am in total and perfect health, now and always." Know that whatever you say is already created, and remember, it is important to speak in the "I am." "I am healthy. I am strong. I am prosperous. I am happy." Speak as though it has already manifested in your life, and speak with enthusiasm.

I used to pray to God asking him to do this and that for me. I bargained with him. I begged him. My results were only fair. When I learned a new way to pray, I began seeing amazing results. I began knowing that God was working in me for perfect health. I didn't have to beg or plead, I just had to know it and it was so. I am convinced that beyond anything, the most important thing I do is my spiritual work. I make the time to do this every day. This is what I believe really healed me.

JUDGE NOT AND PLEASE DON'T GOSSIP

When students begin the Living Foods Lifestyle course, I ask them to not make any judgments about the program until they have completed it. On Day 10 they can draw whatever conclusion they like. What students think on Day 1 is usually completely different by the 10th day. Students who thought they'd never be able to do this program on the first day or two are singing its praises by Day 10. The more Living Foods they eat, the more their bodies want. What seems impossible in the beginning is transformed into the greatest possibility of a lifetime. Things can appear difficult, even impossible, when our brains are full of junk food. When the brain gets real Living Food we think differently. New ideas, hopes, dreams, plans and beginnings will emerge when the brain fog clears.

It's important not to judge something until you have experienced it yourself. It's just as important not to judge other people for where they are and what they do. The only person we have any right to judge is the one we see in the mirror. If you're investigating the raw and Living Foods Lifestyle, you may gather information from many different sources. Some of it may be conflicting information. In this field, as in any other, there are always differences in opinions. I listen to the different views and draw my own conclusions. I may not agree with everything a particular author writes, but I don't discount the entire message. I look for the best I can get out of the message, take that, and leave the rest. Your inner voice will tell you what is the truth and what isn't. You'll find your own answers. The only way to know if something is right for you is to do it, to experience it for yourself. No one can tell you what to do. No one can make the right decisions for you. Know you are greater than you appear to be. Anything is possible when you believe it is. Take charge of your life and let others take charge of theirs.

In addition to eating, gossip is a leading American pastime. There's always someone willing to talk about someone else. Gossiping is harmful and it can be malicious and vicious. It's especially detrimental to the person doing the gossiping, because what goes around comes around. However, it's just as bad for the person who agrees to listen, because listening to gossip adds fuel to the fire. Gossip can hurt others deeply. It can ruin lives. Please don't gossip. My mother always told me, "If they'll talk about someone else to you, then they'll talk about you to someone else." I never forgot this and when people try to gossip to me about others, I stop it dead in its tracks. If you have something to say about someone, say it to him or her – not to someone else.

I remember competing in my first beauty pageant. I was only 16 and there were 15 or 20 other girls competing. Some were my friends, until I won. Then suddenly there were rumors and gossip flying around town about me. Vicious, mean things were said and they hurt, but I refused to let it get me down. I went to one pageant after another, and I won every single time. Pretty soon when I walked in to register for a pageant all the other girls would break up into groups and begin talking about me. They'd talk just loud enough for me to hear. "Well, we might as well go home, there's Miss Aiken, and you know she's going to win. Wonder which judge she's sleeping with?" I was hurt when I heard these things because I was a "good girl" and would never even have thought of sleeping with someone to get anything. I'd go back to my room and cry, until I figured out that crying made my eyes puff up until I looked like a toad. I learned early that people can be cruel, but I kept on going.

In one pageant, another girl wore the same evening dress I did. I couldn't believe it. Of all the evening dresses in all the towns in South Carolina, this girl bought the same dress I did. Pageant officials could have separated us, placing her at one end of the line and me on the other; instead they placed us side by side. I knew they did this on purpose, and the other contestants laughed about it. They said things like, "She deserves it. She thinks she's so great. This ought to knock her down a few notches." It was difficult for me to maintain my composure, smile and act confident but I did, and once again I won.

Pretty soon I had lots crowns and trophies and was the subject of lots of gossip. Was this the price of success? It made what should have been a happy time sad in many ways. However, it taught me much about people and human nature. Generally, people who gossip don't care what they say or who they hurt. If you've ever been the object of malicious gossip, then you know how hurtful it can be. If you've ever been the one gossiping about others, shame on you. I learned that it doesn't really matter what everyone else thinks of you, it matters what you think of yourself. I learned that with success there comes a price.

I learned being a winner can be lonely, but what I gained from competing in those pageants was worth the pain and hurt I endured because I grew and became a better, more confident, more poised young woman. What I learned from this experience was that as long as I believed in myself I could accomplish whatever I set out to do – with or without everyone else's approval. It became important to me to seek out things that would make me happy without trying to please everybody else all the time. I see now that those challenges, and so many other disappointments, were baby steps preparing me for my life today. It prepared me for making the decision to march to a different tune, the Living Foods Lifestyle.

There are always people who try to dissuade others from going after their dreams. There are always those who want to burst another's bubble. There are always those who are jealous of another's success. There are those who gossip about another's life because they don't have a life of their own. There are always mean-spirited, evil, malicious, conniving people trying to put a damper on another's parade or celebration. It doesn't matter, as long as you know you are full of love and you give love and receive love freely.

Wish everyone well, say nothing evil about another and remember everyone is doing the best they can do at the time. Doing so will keep you in God's bubble, where no one or no thing can ever harm you. Make the best decision you can for yourself, no matter what others may say or think. Go after your dream and strive for your goals, even when everyone around thinks you're crazy. Friends and family can sometimes be your worst enemies if they don't agree with your decisions. Be strong.

GOLDEN KEY YOUR TROUBLES AWAY

In his pamphlet, *The Golden Key*, Emmet Fox writes that to "Golden Key" a distressing person or situation will create results in the best interest of all parties.

To "Golden Key" someone or something, speak these words: "I now Golden Key John Doe or Mary Smith or the lawsuit or the bank account." Then say every affirmation you can think of about God. "God is great. God is good. God is all-powerful. God is perfect. God is with me. God is omnipotent. God is love!"

After doing this, forget about the situation until it pops up again, then Golden Key it again. Do this every time a negative situation arises, then step back and watch miracles take place. Relationships will heal. Bank accounts will fill. Pending lawsuits will be cleared up justly to benefit all. Let go, and let God!

A GAME PLAN FOR HEALING

It takes more than just food to help the body heal. I say this again because it's so important. Healing is truly a body-mind-spirit connection. All factors are critical to healing – physical, emotional and spiritual. None can be skipped or ignored. If you're looking for a quick fix, pill or potion, you won't find it in the Living Foods Lifestyle. You must be willing to do the things necessary to obtain good health. Take a look at your lifestyle now. Is it well balanced? Are you making good decisions? Are you taking the time you need for yourself? Are you honoring your spirit?

A number of factors affect healing. When you take responsibility for health and begin to do the most important things, health is restored. Ann Wigmore had four rules to helping us heal; I'll share them with you:

- Eat organic, raw and Living Foods.
- Clean out your colon.
- Stop worrying and relax.
- Expect to heal.

My opinion is that if you reverse these four important steps and start by expecting to heal first, then stop worrying and relax, next, clean out your colon, and of course eat organic raw and Living Foods. You will experience a level of health that is the ultimate high! I encourage you to do it with every bit of positive attitude and energy that you can. Health begins in your mind with the very thoughts you think. If you have been diagnosed with a serious disease, don't claim it. Stop saying things like, "I have cancer." Don't talk in terms of "My cancer." Every time you say that, you reclaim it. Say instead, "I am in perfect health. I am healed." Whatever you say and believe, you will manifest.

CHAPTER
SIX

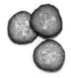

FAVORITE RECIPES

Before giving you these recipes, let me remind you once again that the four main foods, green juices and watermelon juice restore health the quickest. I believe these foods truly helped me heal, and for six months I rarely deviated from them.

In addition to the four main foods for healing, I've included recipes for party and celebration foods. These latter dishes are intended to be used in moderation and to add a little variety to your diet. Rich foods such as these are not the best choice for good health. Even with raw and Living Foods, you can combine poorly or eat too much rich food. That, too, can be a detriment to your health. However, I have found that keeping people motivated on the Living Foods Lifestyle requires varied and tasty dishes. If you are facing a serious health challenge, I recommend a simple diet of green juice, watermelon juice and the four main foods for healing.

Also, I would like to address the salt, fat and sugar issue. Some of these recipes are transitional recipes and are designed to help cooked food eaters get off cooked and go on raw and Living Foods. We are used to greasy, salty and sweet food, and many times just the challenge of changing to uncooked foods can feel overwhelming. So,

I've created recipes with lots of flavor and spice. As you continue on your journey, begin to cut back on the salt, Nama Shoyu, oils, dates and honey. You'll begin to discover the true flavor of foods and you'll soon find you don't want salty, greasy, sweet dishes anymore.

I ate these recipes myself occasionally during my transition process, but now I don't even want to bother with making a recipe. I just eat a piece of fruit or a plate of greens when I'm hungry. My tastes have become very simple. I don't desire rich desserts anymore. It sounds amazing that a sugar addict wouldn't want anything sweet, but all my tastes have changed. I just want fresh, alive fruits and vegetables. It has simplified my life so much, and that has been one of the biggest blessings to me.

Ann Wigmore called the fancier foods Party and Celebration Foods. This implies we should use these foods occasionally, not every day. Just as with cooked foods, raw and Living Food recipes can be poorly combined and too rich for an individual to digest. I think that's why so many people tell me about food they ate at a raw food restaurant that made them sick. These foods, for the most part, are rich, salty and sweet. They taste great, but they can wreak havoc with the digestion. I've experienced the same thing after eating some of these fancy dishes. Listen to your own body. Don't combine too many foods at one time. Don't overeat.

Having said all that, enjoy these wonderful creations that I send to you with love. May they nourish your body, cleanse your mind and heal your spirit.

A LITTLE BIT ABOUT INGREDIENTS

THE BENEFITS OF ORGANIC PRODUCE

I always use organic ingredients, from produce to herbs, spices or anything that goes into my recipes. I may spend a little more money, but the investment in my health is well worth it. Non-organic produce is contaminated by chemicals, sprays and fertilizers. It may have been genetically altered as well. Today, it's difficult to know what you're eating and how safe it is. Genetically altered foods may contain strange combinations – fish cells mixed with strawberries; pig cells mixed with tomatoes – that are not naturally occurring. Genetically altered corn products have made people sick and have even been banned in foreign countries. Buying organic food means no genetic engineering. If you love yourself and your family, you'll insist on organic food whenever possible. Doing so will give you peace of mind, knowing you are doing everything possible to provide you and your family with the most superior food you can find.

If you can grow your own food on good, organic Mother Earth that you have cultivated and nourished with your own hands, that's even better. The more you know about your food, and where it comes from, the better. The type of water used on your crops is equally important because the water becomes part of the food. You may think organic produce is expensive. I have found that not only is it affordable, my food bill has gone down significantly because I'm no longer buying processed, packaged foods. If you've been used to buying meat, dairy and junk food, you will find your grocery bill decreases considerably. Organic is best. You're worth it, and you can afford it. I'd rather spend a little more for good quality food now so I won't have to spend money on prescription drugs and surgery later.

There are those in the raw and Living Foods movement who believe it's more important to eat raw food than all-organic food. Some restaurants use a mix of organic and conventional produce in their recipes. If you believe – as I do – in what Ann Wigmore taught, then you must eat only organic food. If you can't get an organic ingredient, either leave it out, substitute something organic for it, or wait to make the recipe until you can find all-organic components. Peppers, corn and berries are highly sprayed, even more so than other vegetables. If you are eating conventional produce, be aware of the consequences. Organic is best!

THE IMPORTANCE OF WATER

You must stay hydrated. Dehydration is a key factor in disease of the body. Always use good water (be sure you know the source of your water and that it isn't contaminated). Try different waters – charged water, alkaline water and oxygenated water are just a few – and see which works best for you. If you're not sure your water is pure, add a few blades of wheatgrass to it for 15 minutes before using it to help purify, energize and bring life to the water. **Do not use water directly out of the tap, as it may be harmful to your health.** A spring or well of your own, if not contaminated, is one of the best sources of good water. There is so much information out there now about exotic, designer waters. People ask me all the time what I think is best — oxygenated water, charged water, magnetized water, reverse osmosis water, distilled water, etc. I am continually investigating all these waters so I can make a good decision. Currently I use reverse osmosis water and have found it beneficial.

SPROUTING: A HOW-TO GUIDE

Sprouted foods are the cornerstone of the Living Foods Lifestyle. That's why it's called the Living Foods Lifestyle, because the sprouted foods are truly alive! Ann Wigmore's *The Sprouting Book* is a good resource to learn more about sprouting.

Wigmore began sprouting when she acquired an unusual pet, an ailing monkey with no teeth. She tried feeding the monkey seeds but they were too hard, so she put them between wet towels to soften them. The seeds sprouted and she fed them to the monkey who quickly became healthy.

At the same time, Wigmore herself was sick with cancer and other health problems. She had tried eating plain wheatgrass and blended, unsprouted seeds, but it didn't seem to be doing her much good. When she started eating mung bean, sunflower and buckwheat sprouts grown in her own kitchen, she too got well.

Seeds must be soaked before they can sprout. The larger the seed, the more it will expand while soaking. A good rule of thumb is to base soaking times on the size of the seed:

Small Seeds: soak 4 to 6 hours
Medium Seeds: soak 8 to 10 hours
Large Seeds: soak 12 to 24 hours

Soak nuts, seeds, berries, or grains to be sprouted in a glass or stainless steel container (do not use plastic or aluminum). Cover with good, filtered water. Use two or three times as much water as contents; this gives the contents room to expand. Soak for the time recommended in each recipe. Cover the mouth of the container with mesh or cheesecloth and secure with a rubber band. After soaking, drain the water, rinse with fresh water, and drain again. Turn the container at a 45-degree angle and place it on a drain rack. Rinse the contents in the morning and evening with fresh water, each time draining the water off and turning the container on a 45-degree angle. Don't let the contents cover the entire mouth of the container – sprouts need air circulation. When the tail sprouts to approximately the same length as the original berry, seed, grain, or nut, the sprouts are ready. The time this takes will vary with your location, time of year and temperature. Watch the sprouts until the desired length is reached. Use immediately or refrigerate for later use. Sprouts will continue to grow at a slower pace once refrigerated.

A QUICK EXPLANATION OF KITCHEN EQUIPMENT

Having the right machines in the kitchen can make it easier to live the lifestyle and prepare the fabulous recipes to follow. These are some of the machines I like and have found useful.

The Vita-Mix 4500 Turbo is the best high performance blender for making Energy Soup or other soups, salad dressings, sauces, nut and seed cheeses, and nut and seed milks. I have tried other Vita-Mix models, but this one offers the best performance for the best price. I had trouble with other models overheating, which means I had to stop work and put the base of the machine in the freezer to cool it down. This is not convenient. The 4500 model never overheats and I have really put it to the test.

The Omega Juicer is my favorite for juicing fruit and vegetables, grinding nuts, seeds and grains and making numerous specialty recipes. This machine will also juice wheatgrass, which most juicers won't. It does an excellent job and is easy to clean!

The Excalibur Dehydrator is wonderful for dehydrating fruits and vegetables as well as crackers, cookies, breads, pizza, burgers and fruit leathers. It has a temperature control, which is important because some dehydrators without a control are set to dehydrate at 150 degrees or more. When the temperature exceeds 105 degrees, enzymes are destroyed. I prefer the 9-tray dehydrator to smaller models because when I dehydrate, I like to prepare a number of trays of crackers, cookies, etc. Then I can have enough dehydrated foods to last me a few weeks. We set the dehydrators at our Center on 90 degrees because dehydrators tend to run a little hotter than what the thermostat reads.

A Cuisinart Food Processor is a handy timesaver. It's quick

and easy to use for chopping and combining ingredients for many recipes. I prefer the 11-cup size, but there are smaller and larger cup capacities depending on your needs.

The Spiral Slicer is a fun machine that makes angel hair pasta out of vegetables and makes spiral slices for salads and garnishes. My pasta recipes all require the Spiral Slicer, and I love the decorative aspect.

Other Equipment: Sharp knives, a colander, measuring cups and cutting boards are also a must. A variety of wonderful little kitchen gadgets exist to make food preparation fun. Try them and discover what you enjoy and what can help you save time.

When you're preparing food, it's important that your attitude be positive and loving. Why? You transfer your energy into the food and your state of mind affects its taste. Enjoy food preparation and give thanks for the wonderful fruits and vegetables nature has provided. When you share the food you prepare with others, you are sharing a part of yourself.

FOODS FOR HEALING

These foods are easy to prepare, and some of the ingredients are easy to grow right in your own kitchen. Have fun as you watch your food sprout and become full of life. You will feel the energy and become more in touch with Mother Nature. You will detoxify, rebuild and become self-sufficient as you reclaim your health. You will get your power back.

Living this Lifestyle doesn't have to be boring – there are so many wonderful and delicious raw and Living Food recipes besides the four main foods for healing. You can have a ball experimenting. Just remember, whenever you eat, select as many Living Foods as possible. These are the foods that are soaked and sprouted. The more enzyme-rich food you eat, the faster your body will heal. Remember, I ate mostly the four main foods during my first six months, with only occasional fancy recipes. The more disciplined you are, the faster you will progress!

REJUVELAC

Although it's a beverage, Rejuvelac is so nutritious it could be classified as a food by itself. Rejuvelac is the "water" of the Living Foods Lifestyle. Rejuvelac is one of the most important items in the Living Foods Lifestyle because it contains high enzyme levels and helps with digestion. I believe enzyme deficiency is one of the biggest health problems I faced. Rejuvelac helped me restore the enzymes I wasn't getting from cooked food. It also helped remove toxins in my body by providing friendly bacteria in my colon.

Some people are concerned that Rejuvelac and other fermented foods will worsen their yeast or Candida problem. I believe it helped get rid of my Candida and I have seen it help countless others in the same way. In her books, Ann Wigmore maintains that the friendly bacteria in fermented foods such as Rejuvelac, Vege-Kraut and Seed Cheese help get rid of Candida.

As I've mentioned, the two main causes for all disease are toxicity and deficiency of enzymes. Rejuvelac works to overcome these conditions.

- **Toxicity:** A healthy colon is important in eliminating toxins. When our colons are not working properly we become toxic. The healthy bacteria in Rejuvelac and other fermented foods such as Vege-Kraut enable the colon to function properly.
- **Deficiency:** The biggest deficiency most of us face is enzyme deficiency. With its high enzyme levels, Rejuvelac replaces missing enzymes in our bodies, enabling the healing process to take place.

I drink a minimum of eight 8-ounce glasses each day if at all possible. I hated Rejuvelac when I first tried it, but it didn't take me long to start craving it. I'm hooked on Rejuvelac now, and I love the way it tastes.

Rejuvelac is best to drink when it's first made, but it will keep in the refrigerator for a few days. Drink at least eight 8-ounce glasses of Rejuvelac every day. Drink it before you eat to help you digest your food, but avoid drinking any liquids while you are eating. After a meal, wait two hours before drinking if possible. If you absolutely must have something to drink, Rejuvelac is a better choice than water. Rejuvelac is vital in the Living Foods Lifestyle because it is used in so many recipes. It contains vitamin E, so it acts as a natural antioxidant.

In addition to putting enzymes into your body that cooked food doesn't, Rejuvelac helps friendly bacteria such as lactobacillus bifidus grow. Lactobacillus is a natural astringent, which helps the intestines maintain a natural, healthy, vitamin-producing environment. It helps keep the colon clean so fecal waste does not collect on colon walls.

M A K I N G   R E J U V E L A C

- Place 1 cup organic soft spring wheat berries in a wide-mouth glass jar. Cover the mouth of the jar with nylon mesh or a piece of cheesecloth and secure the mesh with a strong rubber band. Add enough spring or filtered water to fill the jar. Allow the wheat berries to soak for 8 to 10 hours, or overnight. After the initial soaking, drain and rinse the berries. Place the jar at an angle on a rack so it can continuously drain. Make sure the wheat berries don't completely cover the mouth of the jar – they need ventilation in order to sprout.
- Rinse the berries about twice a day – morning and evening – while they are sprouting. In about 1½ to 2 days, when the tail is about the same length as the body of the grain, the sprouts are ready to make Rejuvelac. Add spring or filtered water to the sprouted wheat berries and let soak for 48 hours. The ratio for the first batch of Rejuvelac is 3 cups of water to 1 cup of sprouted berries. (This will look like more than the one cup original dry berries because they have plumped up and sprouted tails, but it still counts as 1 cup). After 48 hours, this soaked liquid is your first batch of Rejuvelac. Pour this off into another jar for immediate use or refrigerate for later use.
- Refill the same jar of sprouts with two cups of water for each cup of sprouts. This will make your second batch. Let this batch sit for 24 hours to become Rejuvelac. Pour off this second batch and refill for a third and final batch with 2 cups water for each cup of berries. Again, only 24 hours are needed to make this final batch. After three batches, you can use the berries to make grain crisps, crackers and bread in the dehydrator, or feed them to the squirrels and birds. Do not put them in a compost pile. They will sour the compost because they are fermented.
- Each batch of Rejuvelac will taste slightly different because it is a fermented beverage, made from Living wheat sprouts. Wheat sprouts can vary in their nutritional content, depending on how

long they were sprouted, how often they were rinsed, the type of water used and the temperature they were grown in. Good Rejuvelac is a cloudy, faintly yellow liquid with a tart, lemon-like taste. The best Rejuvelac is slightly carbonated with small bubbles. The length of the tail on the sprout is important. If the sprouts aren't long enough, the Rejuvelac will be weak, and may taste bland or bitter. If the sprouts are too long, it can be too sour or too sweet. It's natural for a layer of white foam to form on top of the Rejuvelac. This is not harmful.

When making Rejuvelac, it's important to rinse the soft wheat berries at least twice daily when they're in the sprouting stage to avoid mold.

ENERGY SOUP

Energy Soup will cleanse and rebuild the body while providing every nutrient you need in a well-balanced, easy-to-digest form. This is important for those suffering from allergies, digestive problems or disease.

Drink an entire blender of Energy Soup throughout the day. For the highest nutritional value, drink your soup during the first 8 to 12 hours after making it. If you have any left, refrigerate it and finish the next day. Energy Soup can be flavored with fresh or dehydrated herbs. My favorites include rosemary, basil and cilantro. Garlic, ginger and cayenne pepper add wonderful flavor and help rid the body of parasites.

If you enjoy other vegetables such as zucchini, celery and cucumbers, add them to the basic mixture. (Just don't leave out any of the main ingredients, which are essential for restoring health.) If you like something crunchy in your soup, add some fresh, finely chopped vegetables on top as a garnish. If you need extra calories, top the Energy Soup with Almond Cream (see recipe on page 143) or put an additional avocado in the mixture.

I N G R E D I E N T S :

- Rejuvelac: Rejuvelac contains vitamins B and E, and more vitamin C than orange juice. It also has valuable, friendly bacteria to help restore the colon to optimum health and plenty of enzymes to aid in digestion. I thought I was allergic to wheat, but found that wheat allergies did not trouble me when I soaked and sprouted the wheat before making Rejuvelac. Soaking and sprouting releases the enzyme inhibitors that give so many people problems with allergies. Grains, seeds and nuts must always be soaked and/or sprouted to release naturally occurring enzyme inhibitors that make the food indigestible. Most people who think they are allergic to wheat have no problem with Rejuvelac. In fact, it helps the body heal.

- **Dulse or Kelp:** These are two of the most nutritious seaweeds in nature, containing all 65 trace elements and minerals, plus plenty of organic iodine.

- **Sprouts:** Mung bean sprouts and lentil sprouts are loaded with enzymes, protein, iron, vitamin C and potassium. They're high in fiber, easy to digest and big energy boosters. Most of all, they are Living Foods because they're sprouted!

- **Greens:** I can't say enough good things about greens. I believe they are one of the most important foods we can eat. They are full of chlorophyll, protein, calcium and so many wonderful nutrients. Choose a variety of greens you like. Kale, collards, chard, dandelion and mustard are all wonderful selections.

- **Buckwheat Sprouts:** These greens are an outstanding source of chlorophyll, vitamin A and C, calcium and lecithin. Lecithin helps eliminate excess cholesterol and cleans out the arteries. These sprouts are excellent for helping the body heal. Buckwheat sprouts are also easy and fun to grow at home.

- **Sunflower Sprouts:** These incredibly nutritious sprouts contain chlorophyll, protein, B complex vitamins, vitamin E, calcium, iron, potassium, magnesium and phosphorus. Like buckwheat, you can easily grow sunflower sprouts at home.

- **Avocado:** Avocados supply vitamin C, A, B1, B2, B3, iron, phosphorus and magnesium. Don't worry about the fat – it's good for you and won't make you fat. If I get a craving for French fries, I eat an avocado and my craving goes away. Many of our cravings are just our bodies wanting more fat. If that happens to you, eat an avocado. It's a delicious way to get added fat and eliminate cravings while nourishing your body.

- **Apples:** Apples mix well with the vegetables in Energy Soup. You might think that combining fruit with vegetables breaks food-combining laws, but relax. When you eat raw and Living Foods you can ease up on some of those laws. Blending apples with the greens in Energy Soup makes both easy to digest. Apples contain protein, fat, carbohydrates, calcium, phosphorus, iron, sodium, potassium, vitamin A, B1, B2, niacin and vitamin C. Ann Wigmore recommends peeling apples because the peels contain enzyme inhibitors, which make them difficult to digest. They can also be waxed. You might think this is OK, but remember my question: "Would you eat a candle?" If you eat waxed fruit, over time you could eat the same amount as in a candle. My mother always told me to eat the skin of apples because that's where all the vitamins are. Actually the vitamins are located right under the skin, so peel thinly. I used to always get stomachaches when I ate apples until I learned about the enzyme inhibitors. Once I began peeling apples, I stopped getting stomachaches. Now they are easy for me to digest.

M A K I N G   E N E R G Y   S O U P

- Place about 1 Tbsp. of **dulse flakes** or **granulated kelp** in a Vita-Mix.
- Fill half the blender with **Rejuvelac**. You can add more when you're finished blending if you want thinner soup. (If you don't have Rejuvelac, use good filtered water.)
- Add ½ cup **sprouted mung beans**, ½ cup **sprouted lentils**, ¼ to 1 peeled, cored and seeded **apple** and blend.
- Add **organic greens** such as chard, kale, mustard, dandelion, arugula, collards, and/or spinach. Fill the blender as full as possible with greens and blend. Add a large handful each of sunflower sprouts and buckwheat sprouts.
- Add ½ to 1 whole **avocado** and finish blending.

VEGE-KRAUT

4 to 6 heads of purple and green **cabbage**
2 oz. chopped **wakame seaweed**, soaked in water for 15 minutes, then drained and cut into bite-size pieces
5 Tbsp. ground **juniper berries**

Remove and save 4 to 6 outer leaves of cabbage. Process the cabbage in the food processor until the juice flows freely. A good way to

135

tell if it's fine enough is to squeeze a handful of cabbage. If the juice flows freely, you know it's OK. If you don't have a food processor and are chopping the cabbage by hand, use a mallet or bat to pound the cabbage until the juice flows. The more the juice flows, the better. I can't stress this enough. If there isn't enough juice coming from the cabbage when you make your kraut, it will be dry and won't ferment properly.

Place an inch and a half layer of purple cabbage in a crock, glass container or stainless steel pot (do not use plastic or aluminum). Place an inch and a half layer of green cabbage on top of that. Press the cabbage down so it is firmly packed. You can use all purple or all green cabbage. Ann Wigmore combined the two to make pink kraut. Sprinkle a tablespoon of ground juniper berries (you can grind them in your Vita-Mix) on top of the cabbage. Cover the layer of cabbage with a light layer of seaweed. Continue layering the ingredients until all the cabbage, juniper berries and seaweed are used. Leave a few inches at the top of the container for expansion as the Vege-Kraut ferments. Cover the contents with the outer cabbage leaves and place a plate atop the leaves. Place something heavy atop the plate (I use a rock) to weigh the contents down. Cover the entire container with a towel or cloth and let sit at room temperature. If you grind your cabbage very fine, three or four days is enough fermentation time because the cabbage is very juicy. If you shredded the cabbage by hand or pounded it with a mallet, it may take up to seven days for fermentation, which happens quicker in a warmer climate.

When the Vege-Kraut is ready, remove the weight, plate and outer leaves. Discard the outer leaves. Juice will be near the surface and sometimes mold will grow on the top during fermentation – this will not hurt you. Just remove and discard the mold. Take a long wooden spoon and insert holes into the mixture so the juice can seep back down into the Vege-Kraut. Mix the contents well. Pack the Vege-Kraut in glass jars and store it in the refrigerator. It will keep anywhere from a few weeks to a few months. Include a cup or more of Vege-Kraut in your daily diet.

OTHER LIVING FOODS MAINSTAYS

FERMENTED FOODS

Fermented foods are important in the Living Foods Lifestyle. The most popular are Rejuvelac, Vege-Kraut and fermented nut and seed dishes, all of which are rich in enzymes, pre-digested protein and lactobacillus bacteria, which improve the intestinal tract and provide an environment to produce vitamins in the intestines. Fermented foods also help constipation problems.

Some people have been told to stay away from fermented foods. You'll have to make your own decision about this, but I don't believe they cause adverse reactions. Toxicity and deficiency inhibit health, not fermented foods. Fermented foods have helped me regain my health.

DEHYDRATED FOODS

Dehydration heats foods slowly at low temperatures so that nutrients and enzymes aren't destroyed. It is important to use a dehydrator with a thermostat. I set mine on 90 degrees. Don't allow the temperature to exceed 105 degrees. You can't always trust that the thermostat is accurate, so check the temperature yourself with a thermometer. When I set my dehydrator to 90 degrees, I am assured that the temperature will not get into the danger zone.

Dehydrated foods are great for snacks or traveling. Dehydrating is practical – you won't ever waste food again. If you're not able to use food in your refrigerator while it's fresh, simply dehydrate it. You can dehydrate most fruits and vegetables. Here are instructions for dehydrating bananas:

- Use ripe bananas – those with brown, speckled skin. They will taste sweeter and have more nutrients.
- Peel the bananas and cut them in half. Cut each half lengthwise to make four strips, or cut in circles if you like.
- Dehydrate for 24 hours, then check to see if they are ready to turn. The fruit should be flexible and leathery.
- Don't dry the fruit until it's excessively hard. Usually one or two days is sufficient. A simple taste test should tell you when it's ready. For chewy bananas, dehydrate 15 to 20 hours. If you like crispy treats, dehydrate 36 to 48 hours.

Try dehydrating any of your favorite fruits or vegetables. Dehydrated vegetables such as corn, peas and carrots make tasty, crunchy snacks. Remember, dehydrated foods are concentrated and should be eaten in moderation. Drink plenty of water when eating concentrated, dehydrated foods. I ate dehydrated foods when I was making the transition from cooked to raw and Living Foods, but now I hardly ever eat anything dehydrated. Dehydrated foods are challenging to digest.

PROTEIN NUGGETS

These tasty treats are easy to make. You'll need:

sunflower seeds (soaked 4 to 6 hours, then drained
  and sprouted for 2 hours)
Rejuvelac
bananas

- Fill the Vita-Mix half full with sunflower seeds and cover with Rejuvelac. Turn on the machine and add bananas until the blender is full. If necessary, add more Rejuvelac to make the mixture easy to blend.
- Pour the batter onto Teflex* sheets and dehydrate for 24 hours.
- Peel nuggets off the Teflex sheets and continue dehydrating on the mesh sheets until the cookies are ready – about 1 to 3 days, less for a chewy nugget, more for a crispy nugget.
- These are great for traveling; just don't eat the entire bag at one sitting.
- Try blending other fruits with sprouted seeds for different cookies.

*Teflex sheets are inserts that go on dehydrator trays. You can pour batter or put wet recipes on these sheets and dehydrate without dripping. They are a must have!

BREAKFAST FOODS

Keep your breakfast light and simple. Give your body and your digestive system time to wake up before eating heavy foods. I drink an ounce of wheatgrass juice upon waking, then I do an enema and wheatgrass implant. After that I go to yoga class or do my yoga exercises at home or in the hotel when I'm traveling. I do not eat until after yoga, and even then I'm not particularly hungry. I drink 16 ounces of Rejuvelac then eat a light meal of fruit if I'm hungry.

SMOOTHIES

Combine alkaline fruits with Rejuvelac and blend in a Vita-Mix until creamy. You can use any fruit you like, but if you have Candida, cancer or diabetes, be careful about eating sweet fruits. Too much fruit is not a good thing for these conditions. In the beginning I hardly ate fruit, but now that I am healed I have added fruit back into my diet in moderation. A simple, easy-to-digest recipe is the apple-avocado smoothie, one of Ann Wigmore's favorites.

APPLE-AVOCADO SMOOTHIE

4 to 6 **apples**, peeled and cored
1 **avocado** (use ½ of an avocado if you are cutting back on fat)
Rejuvelac

* Fill Vita-Mix about ¾ full with apples and avocados.
* Fill the blender to the top with Rejuvelac – less if you want a thicker smoothie. (If you don't have Rejuvelac, use good water.)
* Blend ingredients until creamy and drink.

PAPAYA-MANGO-PINEAPPLE SMOOTHIE

1 **papaya** (peeled and seeded)
1 **mango** (peeled and seeded)
½ **pineapple** (peeled)

Blend in Vita-Mix with a little Rejuvelac or water. This drink makes me think I'm on a tropical island. I love it!

IF YOU HAVE CANDIDA WATCH YOUR FRUIT INTAKE! In the beginning of my health journey, I didn't eat fruit (other than a small amount of apple in the Energy Soup) for six months. This was because I had severe Candida. My Candida healed within six months and I began to add fruit back into my diet. Now I include many fruits in my diet and enjoy them without side effects. You must listen to your own body.

ACID-ALKALINE FORMING FOODS

This is a list of acid-forming and alkaline-forming foods. It must be understood that because a fruit is acid it is no indication that it remains acid in the body. It can turn alkaline. Honey and raw sugar become acid-formers. Those fruits marked with an * should NOT be eaten with any other fruit.

ALKALINE FRUITS

Apples & Cider
Apricots
Avocados
Bananas-yellow
Berries-all
Cantaloupe*
Carob-pod only
Cherries
Citron
Currants
Dates
Figs
Grapes
Grapefruit*
Guavas
Kumquats
Lemons-ripe*
Loquats
Mangos-all
Nectarines
Olives-sundried
Oranges*
Papayas
Passion Fruit
Peaches
Pears
Persimmons
Pineapple-fresh
Plums
Pomegranates
Melons-all*
Prunes
Quince
Raisins
Tamarind
Tangerines

ACID FRUITS

All preserves
Canned-sugared
Cranberries
Dried-sulphured
Glazed Fruits
Olives-Pickles

ALKALINE VEGGIES

Alfalfa
Artichokes
Asparagus
Bamboo Shoots
Beans-green, lima
Beets-all
Broccoli
Cabbage-all
Carrots
Celery
Cauliflower
Chard
Chicory
Coconut
Corn
Cucumber
Dill
Dock
Dulse
Eggplant
Endive
Escarole
Garlic
Horseradish
Jerusalem Artichoke
Kale
Leek
Lettuce
Mushrooms
Okra
Onions
Oyster plant
Parsley
Parsnips
Peppers-sweet
Potatoes
Pumpkin
Radish
Romaine
Rutabagas
Sauerkraut
Soy Bean
Spinach

Squash
Turnips
Water Chestnuts
Watercress

ACID VEGGIES

Asparagus tips
 (white)
Beans-all dried
Brussel Sprouts
Garbanzos
Lentils
Rhubarb

ALKALINE DAIRY

Acidophilus
Buttermilk
Yogurt
Milk-raw only
 (human, cow
 or goat)

ACID DAIRY

Eggs
Butter
Cheese-all
Cream
Custards
Milk-Boiled, cooked,

dried, malted
 or canned

ALKALINE FLESH

Blood and bone
 only and bone
 meal is alkaline

ACID FLESH

All meat, fowl,
 and fish
Gelatin

ALKALINE CEREALS

None (Millet is
 closest
 to neutral)

ALKALINE MISC.

Agar
Coffee Substitute
Honey
Kelp-edible
Tea-herbal

ACID MISC.

Alcoholic Drinks
Coca

Coffee-Indian Tea
All Condiments
Dressings
Drugs
Flavorings
Mayonnaise
Tapioca
Tobacco
Vinegar
Lack of Sleep

ALKALINE NUTS

Almonds
Chestnuts-roasted
Coconut-fresh

ACID NUTS

All nuts except
 those above
Coconut-dried

ACID CEREALS

All Flour Products
All Grains

ONE SHOULD EAT
80% ALKALINE & 20% ACID
FOR BETTER HEALTH.

THESE PERCENTAGES ARE IN THE AMOUNT
OF FOOD EATEN (IN VOLUME).

NUT AND SEED MILK, CREAM AND KEFIR

Many years ago I was a big milk drinker, then I got a kidney stone. The doctor said I was drinking too much milk and eating too much cheese. I cut dairy out of my diet, but I always missed milk – until I began the Living Foods Lifestyle. That's when I learned how to make Almond Milk. It's so delicious and creamy you'll never want cow's milk again. Children love it, too! You can drink it plain or pour on top of Buckwheatie Cereals. This is another recipe I enjoyed during my transition, but don't use anymore. (See recipe for Almond Milk below; Buckwheatie Cereals on page 145.)

In fact, you can make milk out of any nut or seed – sunflower, sesame, almonds, walnuts, etc. First soak the nuts or seeds: 4 hours for small nuts and seeds; 8 hours for medium nuts and seeds and 12 or more hours for large nuts and seeds. Then follow the guidelines for making almond milk and substitute other nuts or seeds of your choice. You can also blend in fruit for flavored milks such as banana, strawberry or peach. Do not use citrus fruits.

To make Kefir, use Rejuvelac when making your milk rather than water. The Rejuvelac ferments the almonds and creates a delicious Kefir. Add just a small amount of Rejuvelac at the time and you can create a thick, rich Kefir without the harmful effects of dairy. Combine fruits to flavor the Kefir, but always listen to your own body, because combining some nuts with fruits can be difficult to digest. Also, I personally don't combine fruits with fats as this combination can promote Candida.

PLAIN ALMOND MILK

1 cup **almonds** (skins off*)
1½ to 3 cups reverse osmosis or filtered **water**, depending
  on desired thickness

- Blend almonds and ½ of the water in the Vita-Mix until the almonds are creamy.
- Add the rest of the water and continue blending. Slowly add water to achieve desired thickness of milk.

*Removing almond skins:
- Place almonds in a stainless steel pot.

- Pour boiling water over the nuts and swish around for 20 to 30 seconds.
- Pour the hot water off and immediately plunge almonds into cold water.
- The skins will easily slip off the almonds just by pinching them between your thumb and forefinger.
- You can make Almond Milk with the skins on the almonds too, but it will be beige, not milky white. Skins can also cause bitterness, so if you leave the skins on, strain the milk through cheesecloth or a sprout bag to get all the skin particles out. This will leave you with rich, creamy milk.

SWEET ALMOND MILK

1 cup **almonds** (skins off)

1½ to 3 cups filtered or spring **water**, depending on desired thickness.

6 Tbsp. **date juice** (this is the soak water poured off dates) or **stevia** (an herbal sweetener that's a safe sugar substitute) to taste. You may add more or less sweetener depending on your taste. You may also blend a couple of dates with the date juice to make a thick, rich sweetener.

1 tsp. **vanilla**

- Follow the Plain Almond Milk recipe above, but add sweetener and vanilla when blending.

CAROB MILK

- Make **Sweet Almond Milk**
- Add ¼ to ½ cup of **raw carob** while blending.
- If you prefer a light milk, cut back on the carob.
- Raw carob is grainier than roasted carob. Sometimes carob will be labeled raw when it's actually lightly roasted. Lightly roasted carob is powdery – like real cocoa powder. It dissolves beautifully, but it's cooked, so don't use it. If in doubt, ask!

ALMOND CREAM

Almond Cream is a way to add variety to Living Foods. It's rich in protein, carbohydrates, calcium, phosphorus, iron, potassium and niacin. It has valuable fat and vitamins B1, B2 and C. Because it's blended with Rejuvelac, it has all the properties of Rejuvelac as well. The stronger the Rejuvelac, the stronger the Almond Cream will taste. Milder Rejuvelac will yield a milder cream. It's rich, so use sparingly. The only difference between Almond Cream and Kefir is that with the Almond Cream you dip the cream off the top, leaving the liquid whey and making a thick cream that will hold its shape. With Kefir you mix in liquid whey to create a smooth, creamy drink.

Use Almond Cream atop Energy Soup or combine with fruits, vegetables, herbs and/or spices to create rich creamy toppings, dressings, yogurt and dips.

> 2 cups **almonds** (soaked for 8 to 12 hours, skins removed*)
> 2 to 3 cups **Rejuvelac**

- Combine almonds and 2 cups Rejuvelac in the Vita-Mix and blend until creamy.
- Add the remaining Rejuvelac if needed and blend until the mixture is smooth.
- Pour the mixture into a glass bowl (no plastic or aluminum). Cover with a cloth and place on a shelf to ferment overnight. Do not refrigerate at this point.
- The next day, spoon the almond cream off the top leaving the liquid whey, which you can drink or save, and blend with the cream for a yogurt drink.
- Use the Almond Cream plain or add herbs and spices to create dips or salad dressings. Place some atop your Energy Soup like sour cream.
- When making dressings or drinks, add whey to give a thinner consistency.

* See instructions for removing almond skins under Plain Almond Milk recipe, page 142.

ALMOND FRUIT KEFIR

> 1 recipe **Almond Cream**
> Extra **whey** to thin the mixture to desired consistency
> **Fruit** of your choice – no citrus

- Blend ingredients in Vita-Mix and enjoy!

BUCKWHEATIE SOFT CEREAL

- Soak hulled buckwheat for about 2 hours then drain the water off and rinse.
- Sprout for 1 to 2 days, rinsing two to three times each day until the sprout is about the same length as the berry.
- Fill the Vita-Mix about ¾ full with peeled apples or other fruit. Add Rejuvelac or water to desired consistency and 1 to 2 cups of sprouted buckwheat. Blend into a creamy cereal and enjoy.
- Experiment by mixing other fruits you like and see if you are able to digest them. Mixing fruit with grains isn't ordinarily a good food combination and I personally wouldn't eat this because I don't eat grains. I did eat them as I was making the transition from cooked food but not anymore. They're too difficult for me to digest. But sprouting the grain and blending with Rejuvelac can help. Listen to your body. If you develop gas or indigestion you'll know this isn't a good combination for you.

CRISPY BUCKWHEATIES

- After sprouting the Buckwheatie Soft Cereal above, place it in a dehydrator and dehydrate until crunchy. This usually takes about 24 to 36 hours.
- Store in an airtight container and when ready to use add Almond Milk and enjoy.
- Sprinkle Crispy Buckwheaties over salads or soups, or just crunch alone.

JUICES

WATERMELON JUICE

Watermelon juice is the most alkaline of any fruit or vegetable, and it can help overcome acidic conditions of the body. It is rich in protein, vitamins A, B, C, enzymes, minerals and chlorophyll, and is easy for most people to digest – even those with poor digestive systems.

It helps eliminate uric acid and dissolve accumulated deposits from a poor diet. I fasted with watermelon juice 10 to 12 times during my first six months and got amazing results. I started out fasting just one or two days at a time. If I felt good I would continue the fast the next day. One of my watermelon juice fasts lasted for 21 days. I felt fabulous afterward. When I fast I drink watermelon juice, green juice and Rejuvelac. I dilute the watermelon juice with Rejuvelac or water so I don't take in too much sugar.

- Peel the outer skin from the melon.
- Juice the entire remaining melon, including the rind, which is the most nutritious part.

KALE-CUCUMBER-CELERY-PARSLEY JUICE

This refreshing juice, which contains chlorophyll, vitamins and minerals, cleanses and helps rebuild the body at a cellular level affecting organs, tissues, muscles and bones. It's full of calcium. This is one of my favorite green juices – I can drink it all day long. It is refreshing and drinking it makes me feel clean and light.

1 bunch **kale**
1 to 2 **cucumbers**
1 to 2 **stalks celery**
1 bunch **parsley**

- Juice all ingredients, mix together and drink.
- If mixture is too green or not sweet enough, add an apple.
- Dilute with Rejuvelac or water if mixture is too concentrated.

LUNCH & DINNER FOODS

BASIC SEED CHEESE

Seed Cheese is a concentrated food and should be used in moderation. It contains good fats, pre-digested protein, B-complex vitamins, vitamin E, calcium, iron, phosphorus, potassium and magnesium. If you're trying to add more calories to your diet, seed cheese is a good choice.

> 1 cup **almonds** (soaked for 8 to 12 hours then drained and rinsed)
> 1 cup **sunflower seeds** (soaked for 8 hours, then drained and sprouted for 8 hours)
> 2 cups **Rejuvelac**
> 3 Tbsp. **wakame seaweed** (hydrated in water)
> 1 Tbsp. **Nama Shoyu raw soy sauce**

- Blend ingredients in Vita-Mix.
- Pour into a muslin cheese bag. You can make a cheese bag easily by using unbleached cotton muslin and sewing it into a bag about 12 to 18 inches wide and deep. If you don't sew, we have wonderful sprout-cheese bags at the Center that are easy to use and easy to clean.
- Place the bag in a colander and place the colander in a bowl to collect the liquid. Cover with a dish towel and allow to ferment 12 to 24 hours in a warm place. The longer you ferment, the stronger the flavor.
- Use plain or add herbs, spices or vegetables to suit your taste.
- Serve with fresh vegetables or use as filler in Nori Rolls, a fresh-tasting mock sushi that's also a raw, Living treat.

NORI ROLL FILLER

Add the following to one recipe of Basic Seed Cheese after it has fermented for 12 to 24 hours:

> 4 Tbsp. raw **tahini**
> 3 Tbsp. **chickpea miso**
> 4 Tbsp. **lemon juice**
> 4 Tbsp. **chopped lemon**
> 4 to 8 **cloves garlic**, finely chopped
> 3 Tbsp. **nutritional yeast**

- Blend all ingredients in the food processor.
- Add Basic Seed Cheese and continue blending until smooth.

NORI ROLLS

- Select raw, sun-dried Nori wrappers (not the toasted ones) and spread cheese mixture in a medium thick layer over ¾ of the Nori wrapper, or put greens and veggies in first and then spread the filling on top of the veggies. This will keep the Nori from getting soggy.
- Fill with sunflower sprouts and thin strips of vegetables such as cucumber, zucchini and carrots.
- Roll tightly and slice in 1½-inch rolls.
- Serve with Nama Shoyu raw soy sauce and wasabi.

BASIC SEED LOAF WITH RED PEPPERS

This is a concentrated food and should be used sparingly.

1 cup **sunflower seeds** (soaked 8 hours and sprouted 4 hours)
½ cup **almonds** (soaked 8 to 12 hours)
½ cup **sesame seeds** (soaked 8 hours)
¼ cup **Rejuvelac** (Don't add this unless you need it to blend. If the peppers are really juicy you won't need the extra liquid.)
6 Tbsp. **wakame seaweed**
1 Tbsp. **Nama Shoyu raw soy sauce**
6 to 8 **cloves garlic**
1 large **red pepper**

- Drain nuts and seeds completely – leftover water will result in a soupy mixture. Juice from the red pepper can also cause soupiness, so judge for yourself how much to add.
- Place all ingredients in the food processor and mix until the seeds are ground up and the texture is smooth.
- Place into a bowl or pat into a loaf and refrigerate overnight to ferment. The longer it sets, the stronger the flavor becomes.
- Eat alone, stuff into celery stalks or red peppers, or use as filler for Nori Rolls.
- You can ferment this for 4 to 6 hours outside the refrigerator for a stronger, more pungent taste.

LIVING HUMMUS

1 cup **garbanzo beans** soaked for 12 hours and sprouted for 24 hours (Don't over sprout; this can cause a bitter taste.)
4 to 5 large **garlic cloves**
$^1/_3$ cup **lemon juice**
$^1/_3$ cup **olive oil**
3 Tbsp. **chickpea miso**
1 tsp. **dried jalapeno pepper** or 2 Tbsp. **fresh jalapeno**
3 Tbsp. **raw tahini**

- Chop garlic and jalapeno pepper in food processor.
- Add drained garbanzo beans and blend.
- Add lemon juice, miso, tahini, half the olive oil and blend.
- Add remaining olive oil and blend to a creamy consistency.
- For good food combining, eat hummus with fresh vegetables, not crackers.

WALNUT STEAK

2 cups **walnuts** (soaked 8 hours)
1 cup **sunflower seeds** (soaked 8 hours)
1 cup **almonds** (soaked 8 hours)
6 **cloves garlic**
1 tsp. **Celtic sea salt**
$^1/_2$ cup **onion**
2 Tbsp. fresh **rosemary**
1 cup **red bell pepper**
1 Tbsp. **dried jalapeno pepper** or 3 Tbsp. if **fresh pepper** (adjust peppers according to taste)
$1^1/_2$ tsp. **cumin powder**
2 cups fresh **tomatoes**
1 cup **sun-dried tomatoes** (soaked 1 to 2 hours then drained)
9 **dates** (soaked 1 to 2 hours)
6 fresh **basil leaves** or 1 tsp. **dried basil**

- Mix garlic, salt, onion, rosemary, red pepper, jalapeno pepper, cumin, tomatoes, dates and basil in food processor.
- Blend nuts in processor.

- Continue blending until the texture is smooth.
- Form into 4 to 5 ounce patties or one large loaf and dehydrate for 2 hours.
- Serve warm or make ahead of time, refrigerate and serve cold.
- You can use as a dip or spread if you don't dehydrate.

SPICY WALNUT TOMATO PATÉ

4 cups **walnuts** (soaked 8 hours)
8 **cloves garlic**
1 Tbsp. **Nama Shoyu** raw soy sauce
1 cup **onion**
1 cup **red bell pepper**
2 Tbsp. **dried jalapeno pepper** or 6 Tbsp. if **fresh pepper** (adjust peppers according to taste)
1½ tsp. **cumin powder**
3 cups fresh **tomatoes**
6 **dates** (soaked for 1 to 2 hours)
½ cup **fresh cilantro** or 1 Tbsp. **dried cilantro**

- Blend garlic, salt, onion, cilantro, red bell pepper, jalapeno pepper, cumin, tomatoes, dates and basil in the food processor.
- Add nuts and blend until smooth.
- Serve with fresh vegetables or crackers.

VEGGIE NUT SEED LOAF

1 cup **almonds** (soaked 8 to 12 hours)
½ cup **sunflower seeds** (soaked 8 hours, sprouted 4 hours)
½ cup **sesame seeds** (soaked overnight, sprouted 4 hours)
⅓ cup **Rejuvelac**
½ cup **red bell pepper**, minced
½ cup **parsley**, minced
½ cup **celery**, minced
½ cup **onions**, minced
1 Tbsp. **Nama Shoyu** raw soy sauce
6 Tbsp. **wakame seaweed** (hydrated in water for 20 minutes, then drained)
1 cup **fresh basil** or 2 Tbsp. **dried basil**

- Blend almonds, sunflower seeds, sesame seeds, Rejuvelac, Nama Shoyu raw soy sauce, fresh basil and wakame in food processor until the nuts and seeds are combined.
- Mince vegetables by hand, not in the food processor, so they will be small and chunky.
- Hand mix the nut seed mixture with the vegetables and refrigerate overnight to ferment. Or, leave the mixture out at room temperature for 4 to 6 hours for a more fermented taste. Divide the recipe and ferment half in the refrigerator and the other half on the kitchen counter so you can taste the difference.

GARBANZO SUNFLOWER LOAF

3 cups **garbanzo beans** (soaked overnight
   and sprouted 24 hours)
½ cup **sesame seeds** (soaked 8 hours, sprouted 4 hours)
1 cup **sunflower seeds** (soaked 8 hours, sprouted 4 hours)
1 cup **onion**, chopped
1½ cup **celery**, chopped
½ cup **red bell pepper**, chopped
4 **cloves garlic**, minced
4 Tbsp. fresh **cilantro**
4 Tbsp. **lemon juice**
½ tsp. **Celtic sea salt**
1 tsp. **cayenne pepper**
2 Tbsp. **chickpea miso**
2 Tbsp. **raw tahini**

- Chop garlic and cilantro in food processor.
- Add lemon juice, sea salt, cayenne pepper, miso and tahini then blend.
- Add garbanzo beans, sesame seeds and sunflower seeds; continue blending until smooth.
- Remove from the food processor and fold in onion, celery and red bell pepper.
- Form into a loaf and dehydrate for 2 to 4 hours, or longer. The longer you dehydrate the loaf, the drier it will become.
- Drizzle with Hot Curry Sauce (see recipe on page 158) and serve with Veggie Sprout Relish Salad (see recipe on page 162).

NUTTY LENTIL BURGERS

2 cups **sprouted lentils** (see page 128 for sprouting directions)
½ cup **sesame seeds** (soaked 8 hours, sprouted 4 hours)
1 cup **sunflower seeds** (soaked 8 hours, sprouted 4 hours)
1 cup **almonds** (soaked 8 hours, sprouted 4 hours)
1½ cups **onion**, chopped
1 cup **red bell pepper**, chopped
6 **cloves garlic**, minced
1 cup **fresh basil**
2 Tbsp. **lemon juice**
½ tsp. **Celtic sea salt**
2 Tbsp. fresh **jalapeno pepper**
3 Tbsp. **chickpea miso**

- Chop garlic in the food processor.
- Add basil and jalapeno; continue chopping.
- Add garbanzo beans, sesame seeds, sunflower seeds and almonds; continue processing until well blended.
- Add lemon juice, sea salt and miso; continue blending.
- Remove from food processor and fold in onion and red pepper.
- Form into individual burgers.
- Dehydrate for 2 to 4 hours or longer, depending on the texture you like. The longer you dehydrate the patties, the drier and chewier they will become.
- Serve on lettuce leaves, garnish with sliced onion and tomato.

DESSERTS

COCONUT ALMOND TRUFFLES

2 cups **almonds** (soaked 8 hours, sprouted 4 hours)
1 cup **dried coconut**
3 cups **pitted dates** (soaked 4 hours)
½ cup **date juice** (from soaking dates)
Extra **coconut** to roll the balls in

- Blend almonds in the food processor until finely chopped.

- Add dates, coconut and date juice (only if needed) to form dough-like consistency. You may not need any additional juice if the dates are juicy enough. You want the mixture to hold together in a ball, so it can't be soupy.
- When fully blended, roll into balls, then roll balls into coconut.
- Refrigerate 2 hours or more to set.

CAROB-RAISIN TRUFFLES

2 cups **almonds** (soaked 8 hours)
3 cups **raisins** (soaked 4 hours)
2 cups **pitted dates** (soaked 4 hours)
$^1/_2$ to $^3/_4$ cups **raw carob** (adjust according to taste)
$^1/_2$ cup **raisin or date juice** (from soaking raisins and dates)
Extra **carob** to roll the balls in

- Blend almonds in food processor until finely chopped.
- Add carob, dates, raisins and raisin juice or date juice. Process lightly so raisins are still in chunks.
- Form into balls and roll in carob.
- Refrigerate to set.

ALMOND SUNFLOWER DATE PIE CRUST

Makes 1 thick crust or 2 thin crusts

2 cups **almonds** (soaked overnight – they will expand)
1 cup **sunflower seeds** (soaked overnight)
1 cup **soaked dates***
* Check dates before placing in food processor to be sure pits are removed.

- Chop nuts and seeds first in food processor.
- Add dates and continue processing until well blended.
- Press the blended mixture into one or two glass pie plates.
- Set dehydrator on 90 degrees and dehydrate overnight for a crunchy crust.
- Add any raw pie filling you like.
- Use this mixture to make cookies. Form into cookie shapes and dehydrate until chewy or crunchy, whichever you like best.

APPLE MOUSSE PIE FILLING

5 **apples** (peeled, cored and cut in chunks)
1 cup **dates** pitted and soaked overnight (save the soak juice)
⅓ cup **raisins** (soaked overnight)
¾ tsp. **cinnamon**
1 Tbsp. **psyllium seed powder**

- Place all ingredients, except psyllium, in the food processor and blend until smooth.
- Add psyllium a little at a time after the mixture is completely smooth.
- For mousse, place filling in bowl and serve plain, or top with macadamia cream and sprinkles of almond date crust.
- For pie, line the bottom of the piecrust (see recipe on page 153) with thin slices of apple. Cover apples with filling and refrigerate for 2 hours before slicing. Serve plain or with Macadamia Cream Topping (see recipe below).

MACADAMIA CREAM TOPPING

1 cup **macadamia nuts** (soaked overnight)
10 **pitted dates** (soaked overnight)
5 Tbsp. **date juice** (from soaking water)
¾ tsp. **vanilla**

- Grind nuts in food processor.
- Add dates and date juice and continue blending.
- Transfer to the Vita-Mix and add more date soak water. Blend until smooth and creamy.
- Use as a topping for desserts or shape into cookies and dehydrate.

YAMMY PIE

1 recipe Almond-Sunflower-Date piecrust

Filling:
1½ cup **dates** (pitted, soaked 4 hours, reserve soak water)

2 cups **yams** peeled and cut in chunks
6 Tbsp. **date juice** (reserved from soaking dates)
1¹/₂ tsp. **cinnamon**
¹/₄ tsp. **vanilla**
¹/₂ tsp. **Chinese 5-spice powder**
¹/₄ tsp. **mace**
1 Tbsp. **psyllium powder**

- Grind yams in the food processor.
- Add remaining ingredients, except psyllium. Blend until smooth.
- Gradually add psyllium with processor running.
- Pour filling into the crust immediately.
- Refrigerate for 2 hours before serving.
- Serve plain or top with macadamia cream.

BANANA STRAWBERRY ICE CREAM

- Peel **bananas**, wash **strawberries** and freeze.
- Alternate bananas and strawberries through the Omega Juicer for a beautiful, swirled ice cream.
- Choose other fruits you like to create an array of refreshing and delicious ice creams and sorbets. Kids love this.

SALAD DRESSINGS, SAUCES & DIPS

GARLIC-DILL DIP

1 recipe **Almond Cream** (see recipe on page 143)
3 Tbsp. **dried dill** or ³/₄ to 1 cup **fresh dill**, depending on
   your taste
¹/₂ tsp. **Celtic sea salt** (add more if taste is bland)

- Mix ingredients by hand, in the food processor or Vita-Mix.
- Refrigerate overnight.
- Serve with fresh veggies or crackers.

155

CREAMY RANCH DRESSING

1 recipe **Almond Cream** (see recipe on page 143)
¹/₂ to 1 cup **whey** (This liquid will separate when making almond cream and will go to the bottom of the bowl.)
3 **cloves garlic**, minced
3 **green onions**, chopped (include green tops)
¹/₂ tsp. **dried dill**
¹/₂ tsp. **dried basil**
¹/₂ tsp. **dried thyme**
¹/₂ tsp. **Celtic sea salt** (may require more if taste is bland)
(If you use fresh herbs instead of dried, increase measurement to 2 Tbsp.)

- Mix all ingredients in the Vita-Mix.
- Add just enough whey to give dressing the desired consistency.

GINGER GARLIC PEPPER SALAD DRESSING

1 tsp. **cayenne pepper**
¹/₄ cup **garlic**, chopped
2 Tbsp. **fresh ginger**
1 Tbsp. **Nama Shoyu raw soy sauce**
3 Tbsp. **raw tahini**
¹/₂ cup **lemon juice**
1 cup **olive oil**

- Place all ingredients in Vita-Mix and blend.

CREAMY SWEET ALMOND DRESSING

1 cup **almond cream**
¹/₂ cup **date juice** or **stevia** (an herbal sweetener) to taste

- Mix in Vita-Mix and serve over fruit.

TOMATO PEPPER DRESSING

6 cups **fresh tomatoes**
4 **cloves garlic**

1 red bell pepper
1 jalapeno pepper if fresh (if dried pepper use 1 tsp.)
3 lemons, juiced
1 tsp. Celtic sea salt
2 cups olive oil

- Place ingredients (except oil) in Vita-Mix.
- Add half the oil and blend.
- Slowly add remaining oil. (This gives a creamy texture. If you add the oil too fast it will separate and not be creamy.)

SUNNY SIDE DRESSING

Juice of 5 lemons
5 cloves garlic
2 Tbsp. fresh ginger
2½ cups tomatoes
1 cup carrots
½ tsp. Celtic sea salt or 1 Tbsp. Nama Shoyu raw soy sauce
¾ cup olive oil
¼ to ½ cup water

- Place ingredients in Vita-Mix and blend until creamy.

TOMATO BASIL SAUCE

3 cups fresh tomatoes
3 cups sun-dried tomatoes (soaked 1 to 2 hours, then drained)
1½ cup fresh basil (3 Tbsp. if dried)
4 cloves garlic, chopped
3 Tbsp. lemon juice
1 tsp. Celtic sea salt
3 Tbsp. olive oil
9 dates* (soaked 1 to 2 hours and drained)
* Check dates before placing in food processor to be sure pits are removed.

- Place garlic in food processor and chop.
- Add dates and blend well.
- Add sun-dried tomatoes and blend.

- Add remaining ingredients and blend until smooth.
- Use immediately or refrigerate overnight so flavors meld together.

CURRIED LENTIL DIP

>4 cups **sprouted lentils**
>   (see page 128 for sprouting directions)
>1 cup **onion**, chopped
>1 cup **red bell pepper**, chopped
>1 cup **Hot Curry Sauce** (see recipe below)

- Mix sprouted lentils, onion and red pepper in a bowl.
- Add 1 cup of Hot Curry Sauce and blend.
- This makes a chunky dip. If you like a creamier dip, place ingredients in the food processor or Vita-Mix; blend until your dip reaches the desired consistency.

HOT CURRY SAUCE

>3 oz. **date juice** and **blended, soaked dates***
>½ cup **lemon juice**
>⅔ cup **garlic**
>2 cups **macadamia nuts** (soaked overnight and drained)
>3 tsp. **Celtic sea salt**
>2 Tbsp. **fresh ginger**
>1 Tbsp. **turmeric**
>6 Tbsp. **curry powder**
>6 small **fresh jalapeno peppers**. If **dried jalapeno** use 2 Tbsp.
>3 cups **onion**
>3 tsp. **cayenne pepper**
>2 cups **olive oil**
>1 to 1½ cups **water**
>* Soak and blend 4 pitted dates (save soak juice).

- Blend well in the Vita-Mix, adding water in small amounts until your sauce reaches the desired consistency.
- This makes a thick sauce that can be used for a dip or diluted with water for a salad dressing.
- This sauce is rich, hot and spicy, so use sparingly.

SALADS

CURRY CABBAGE LENTIL SALAD

4 cups **chopped cabbage** (purple, green or a
   combination of each)
2 cups **sprouted lentils** (see page 128 for sprouting
   directions)
1 Tbsp. **curry powder**
½ cup **onion**, chopped
4 **cloves garlic**, chopped
½ cup **red bell pepper**, chopped
4 Tbsp. **lemon juice**
¼ cup **olive oil**
1 tsp. **Celtic sea salt**

- Combine curry powder, garlic, lemon juice, olive oil and Celtic sea salt.
- Chop onions and red pepper, then combine with cabbage and lentils.
- Cover with dressing and toss well.
- Marinate in refrigerator; the flavors will blend best if left overnight.
- For more spice and zip add ½ to 1 cup Hot Curry Sauce (see recipe on previous page).

COMPLETE MEAL SALAD FOR TWO

The Complete Meal Salad for Two includes protein, carbohydrates, minerals, vitamins and enzymes in sufficient quantity and quality to furnish excellent energy to the body, along with the elements needed for growth or maintenance. Fresh, raw, organic garden vegetables, sprouts and seeds are rich in vitamins, minerals and enzymes. A little dulse or kelp seaweed adds flavor and minerals. This is a complete meal in every way. Add one of your favorite salad dressings for different tastes.

½ cup **sunflower sprouts greens**
½ cup **buckwheat lettuce sprouts greens**

1 cup **mung bean sprouts** (see page 128 for sprouting
  directions)
1 cup **summer squash** or **zucchini**, grated or chopped
1 cup **mixed greens** (kale, spinach, arugula, collards
  or your choice of favorite greens)
½ **avocado**, sliced
¼ **cucumber** sliced (if the cucumber is waxed, peel first)
4 slices **red bell pepper**
2 Tbsp. **sunflower seeds** (soaked 8 hours, sprouted
  8 hours)
2 Tbsp. **coconut oil**
1 Tbsp. **kelp** (granulated) or dulse (flakes)

- Toss ingredients in a bowl and serve immediately.

CUCUMBER TOMATO SALAD

2 **cucumbers** peeled and chopped into medium, bite-sized
  chunks
4 **small tomatoes** chopped into medium, bite-sized chunks
1 Tbsp. **minced garlic**
1 cup **onion**, chopped fine
1 tsp. **Nama Shoyu raw soy sauce**
¼ cup **sesame oil**
¼ cup **lemon juice**

- Toss ingredients in a bowl and serve immediately.
- Or, let marinate overnight to enhance flavor.

FRESH TOMATO, BASIL
AND PINE NUT SALAD

12 **Roma tomatoes**, chopped
1 cup **pine nuts** (soaked for 30 minutes, then drained)
1½ cups **fresh basil**, chopped
½ tsp. **Celtic sea salt**
Cayenne pepper to taste

- Mix ingredients together and enjoy as a salad, or place atop
  Raw Zucchini Pasta (see recipe on page166).

HIZIKI CABBAGE SALAD
WITH TOMATOES AND GARLIC SESAME SAUCE

1/2 cup **Hiziki seaweed** (soaked in water for 30 minutes, then drained)

1/2 cup **onion**, finely chopped

4 cups chopped **cabbage** (mixture of green and/or purple)

1 Tbsp. **dried jalapeno peppers** or 4 Tbsp. **fresh jalapeno peppers**

1/2 cup **lemon juice**

1/4 cup **sesame oil**

1 Tbsp. **tahini**

1 tsp. **Nama Shoyu raw soy sauce**

2 Tbsp. **garlic**, chopped

1 cup **tomatoes**, chopped

- Mix seaweed, cabbage, onion and tomatoes together in a large bowl.
- Blend jalapeno peppers, lemon juice, sesame oil, tahini, Nama Shoyu and garlic in the food processor or Vita-Mix. Blend until creamy, then pour over the vegetable mixture.
- Mix well and marinate overnight. You can serve immediately, but marinating blends the flavors and makes the dish taste richer.

SEAWEED CUCUMBER SALAD

1 bag mixed, dried **seaweed salad** (This comes pre-packaged in health food stores.
I have used two brands, Sokin and Eden.
You can also use other dried seaweeds of your choice.)

2 **cucumbers** peeled and sliced thin

8 Tbsp. **lemon juice**

1 Tbsp. **Nama Shoyu raw soy sauce**

4 Tbsp. **sesame oil**

1 **onion**, chopped fine

1 **red pepper**, chopped fine

4 large **cloves garlic**, minced fine

- Mix all ingredients together and serve.
- If refrigerated, this dish will keep 3 to 5 days. The flavors will blend more fully as it sits.

VEGGIE SPROUT RELISH SALAD

2 cups **fresh tomatoes**, chopped
1½ cups **zucchini**, chopped
1 **avocado**, chopped
Juice of ½ **lemon**
2 **cloves garlic**, minced
1 **jalapeno pepper**, seeded and chopped
1 tsp. **Nama Shoyu raw soy sauce** to taste
2 cups **clover sprouts**

- Mix ingredients, except sprouts, together to make a relish.
- Top with 2 cups clover sprouts.

MARINATED GREENS

5 cups **kale** or **dark leafy greens** of your choice
⅓ cup **carrots**, finely chopped
⅓ cup **zucchini**, finely chopped
⅓ cup **red pepper**, finely chopped
1 to 2 Tbsp. **garlic**, chopped
½ cup **lemon juice**
½ cup **Nama Shoyu raw soy sauce**
½ **cup oil** (sesame, olive or flax – choose the one you like the best)

- Choose the greens you like best. You may use one type alone or you may mix the greens. Some good choices include kale, collards, dandelion and mustard.
- Chop greens and other vegetables into small pieces so they will digest easier. You can do this by hand or in the food processor.
- Place all ingredients into a bowl and toss well, until the liquid completely coats the greens. Refrigerate and marinate 2 to 24 hours before serving. The longer it marinates, the richer the flavor becomes.

- For more marinade, double the amounts of sesame oil, Nama Shoyu and lemon juice.

APPLE WALDORF SALAD

4 cups **apples**, peeled, cored and cut into bite-sized pieces
2 cups **celery**, chopped into bite-sized pieces
1 cup **walnuts** (soaked 8 hours)
1 cup **raisins** (soaked 4 hours)

- Combine nuts and fruits together and enjoy as is.
- Or add Creamy Sweet Almond Dressing (see recipe on page 156) for a more traditional Waldorf salad.
- Add $1/2$ cup date cream (made by blending 4 soaked dates with $1/2$ cup soak water until creamy).

SWEET POTATO SALAD

5 cups **sweet potatoes**, cut into bite-sized pieces
$3/4$ cup **dates**, soaked 4 hours and chopped into
    bite-sized pieces
$3/4$ cup **walnuts**, soaked 8 hours and chopped
$1/2$ cup **date juice** (from soaking dates)
$3/4$ Tbsp. **cinnamon**

- Combine all ingredients, toss and serve.

CRACKERS & COOKIES

FIESTO CRACKERS

2 cups **sunflower seeds** (soaked 8 hours)
2 cups **walnuts** (soaked 8 hours)
2 cups **almonds** (soaked 8 hours)
12 Tbsp. **flax seeds** (soaked 30 minutes in water 1 inch over seeds)
2 cups chopped **fresh tomato**
2 cups **onion**, chopped
2 Tbsp. **cumin powder**
1 tsp. **Celtic sea salt**
3 tsp. **dried jalapeno peppers** or 3 Tbsp. **fresh jalapeno peppers**

- Place jalapeno peppers, tomato and onion in food processor and blend until creamy.
- Add drained seeds and nuts, cumin and sea salt and continue blending until all ingredients are mixed well and the nuts are finely chopped. The batter should be creamy and easy to spread.
- Spread mixture on Teflex dehydrator sheets. Make thick or thin crackers, depending on how much mixture is spread on each sheet. Usually 1 recipe makes 2 Teflex sheets.
- Dehydrate at 90 degrees overnight. The next day flip the crackers and peel off the Teflex sheet, leave on the mesh sheet and continue dehydrating until crispy. This should take 24 to 36 hours. To test the crackers, break off a piece and see if it's crunchy enough for your taste.

MEXI-CRISP CRACKERS

$^1\!/_2$ cup **sun-dried tomatoes** (soaked 1 to 2 hours, then drained) or 1$^1\!/_2$ cups **fresh tomatoes**
2 **cloves garlic**
$^1\!/_2$ cup **onion**
$^1\!/_2$ tsp. **Celtic sea salt**
2 Tbsp. **dried jalapeno pepper** or 6 Tbsp. **fresh jalapeno peppers**
2 Tbsp. **date juice** (from soaking 3 to 4 dates)
2 tsp. **cumin powder**
6 cups **Rejuvelac berries** or **sprouted soft wheat berries** (if you use Rejuvelac berries – the soft wheat berries that remain after the third, and final, batch of Rejuvelac – the crackers will have a sour taste. Sprouted soft wheat berries give a sweeter taste.)

- Combine all ingredients in a food processor and blend.
- Spread on dehydrator sheets and dehydrate at 90 degrees overnight.
- Flip the crackers over the next day and continue dehydrating until crispy. This could take up to 2 days.
- Break into crackers and store in an airtight container.

ONION CRACKERS

2 cups **onion**
1 tsp. **Celtic sea salt**
6 Tbsp. **date juice** (from soaking 3 to 4 dates)
6 cups **Rejuvelac berries** or **sprouted soft wheat berries***
* See Mexi-Crisp Crackers, page 164, for information on
   Rejuvelac berries vs. soft wheat berries.

- Chop onion in food processor. Add berries and blend until chopped. Add Celtic sea salt and date juice. Blend well.
- Spread onto dehydrator sheets and dehydrate overnight at 90 degrees.
- Flip the crackers over the next day and continue dehydrating until crispy.
- For a chewy cracker, dehydrate less; for a crispy cracker, dehydrate longer.
- Break into crackers and store in an airtight container.

NUTTY DATE COOKIES

1 cup **almonds** (soaked 8 hours)
1 cup **walnuts** (soaked 8 hours)
1 cup **sunflower seeds** (soaked 8 hours)
2 cups **soaked dates*** (soaked 4 hours)
* Check dates before placing in food processor
   to be sure pits are removed.

- Chop nuts and seeds thoroughly in the food processor.
- Add dates and continue processing until well blended. For chunky cookies, process for a shorter time.
- Form into cookies on Teflex sheets and place into dehydrator overnight at 90 degrees.
- Check cookies after 12 hours, turn them and continue to dehydrate.
- Dehydration time depends on your choice of moist, chewy cookies or crispy, crunchy cookies. Try different dehydration times to see which you like best.

MACADAMIA-ALMOND-DATE COOKIES

2 cups **macadamia nuts** (soaked overnight)
1 cup **almonds** (soaked overnight)
20 **pitted dates** (soaked overnight)
5 Tbsp. **date juice** (from the soaking water)
¾ tsp. **vanilla**

- Place nuts in food processor and grind – leave them chunky.
- Add dates and date juice, continue processing until the mixture holds together.
- Form into cookies and dehydrate at 90 degrees until chewy or crunchy (24 to 48 hours).

RAW PASTAS

You can use any salad dressing recipe as a topping for pasta.

RAW ZUCCHINI PASTA

8 cups **zucchini** (sliced in the spiral slicer on the
angel hair setting)
1 to 2 cups **Tomato Basil Sauce** (see recipe on page 157)

- Spiral slice zucchini into angel hair pasta noodles.
- Cut noodles so they are not one continuous string.
- Add as much Tomato Basil Sauce as you like and toss; be sure all noodles are coated.
- For a garnish, top with Fresh Tomato, Basil Pine Nut Salad (see recipe on page 160).

CHAPTER
SEVEN

CLOSING THOUGHTS

WHAT NEXT?

Now that you have some information about the Living Foods Lifestyle, what will you do with it? Knowledge is power, but it's also responsibility. What responsibility will you take for your own health and your life?

No matter what you decide, remember this is your own personal journey. There's no competition or race going on among Living Foodists. If you choose to do this, do it for yourself, not because you're competing with someone else or trying to please someone else. We honor everyone on his or her individual path, and we understand that everyone must make decisions about how much, if any, of this Lifestyle to put into practice.

If you do decide to embrace the Living Foods Lifestyle, you're in store for a wonderful journey. It has made a tremendous difference in my life and in the lives of many others. Even if you only add a small percentage of Living Foods to your diet, you will be getting more enzymes, vitamins and minerals than probably ever before. Start where you are, as small or big as you like – just start. As you feel the wonderful effects of Living Foods, you may do what so many others have done and add more and more into your diet.

Some students don't think they'll ever be able to live this Lifestyle 100 percent. But after learning to prepare the foods and trying it for 10 days, they say, "I'll do this for the rest of my life – it makes me feel so good." No matter what percentage of Living Foods you decide to continue to add to your diet, you will reap benefits. Begin where you are and proceed at your own pace.

I hope this book helps start you on your course to a healthy lifestyle. If you're like me, hands-on training will help you understand how to do everything properly. I learn more by doing than just reading. If that's the case, please join us at the Living Foods Institute in Atlanta, Georgia, or Miami Beach, Florida, for our 10-Day Living Foods Lifestyle Course. You'll get the practice you need with hands-on training in the kitchen and the support and encouragement you need to stay focused on the results you want. Not only will you learn how to prepare the foods, you'll learn exactly what to do each day to help your body, mind and spirit to heal.

I wish each of you who are on the journey for health and happiness much success. I said earlier that knowledge is power. More important – **knowledge is responsibility.** Take responsibility for your health and make nutritional and lifestyle changes today that will benefit you for a lifetime. You're worth it!

THE 10-DAY LIVING FOODS LIFESTYLE COURSE

The 10-Day Living Foods Lifestyle Course is designed to teach you delicious healing recipes and the body-mind-spirit connection to healing. We designed our program to be both comprehensive and empowering. We want you to know what you're doing when you complete this course. The 10-Day Program is offered for 10 consecutive days. If you can't come for 10 straight days, you can make up classes during the first four months from the date you sign your training agreement. Call our Center for a list of upcoming dates and availability. Here's an overview of what awaits you each day:

You'll enjoy a delicious, nutritious organic Living Foods meal including the four main foods for healing and gourmet Living Foods recipes.

You'll learn lessons on detoxification and rebuilding your body, mind, and spirit on every level from food combining to exercise and essential oils.

You'll take part in a powerful emotional and spiritual healing class designed to help you forgive, release the past and move with ease to the next level so you can realize authentic power, fulfillment, joy and happiness in your life.

MATERIAL COVERED DURING 10-DAY TRAINING

This is a partial list of what you will learn:

Day 1 What is the Living Foods Lifestyle?
The Four Most Important Foods for Healing
The Nutritional Value of Energy Soup, Rejuvelac,
   Wheatgrass and Vege-Kraut
Growing Wheatgrass, Buckwheat and Sunflower Sprouts
Soaking Seeds and Grains

The Nature of Disease and Symptoms
The Solution to the Health Problems that Plague Our Society
The Right Attitude for Healing
Change Your Mind and Change Your World
Recipe – Cucumber Tomato Salad
Recipe – Rejuvelac
Recipe – Marinated Greens
Recipe – Young Coconut Smoothie

Day 2 Sprouting Berries, Grains and Seeds
Enzymes in Living Foods
Enzymes and Medical Research
Enzymes and Weight Control
Overeating and Weight Management
Food Combining
Never Be Hungry with Living Foods
Fasting for Health
Detoxification, A Must to Achieve Health
Healing Crisis: Are You in One?
Colon Health – All Disease Begins in the Colon
Recipe – Zucchini Carrot Dill Salad
Recipe – The Complete Meal Salad
Recipe – Tomato Pepper Dressing

Day 3 The Contents of Wheatgrass
Wheatgrass Juicing
Wheatgrass and Its Miracles
How to Plant and Grow Wheatgrass, Buckwheat and
   Sunflower Sprouts
Wheatgrass Implants and Their Power to Heal
35 Uses for Wheatgrass
The Food Basics – What to Eat and When
Blending Foods for Better Digestion
Recipe – Energy Soup
Recipe – Vege-Paté
Recipe – Tara Country Club Salad

Day 4 Toxicity and Deficiency
Detox Symptoms and How to Make Detoxing Easier
Benefits of Fermented Foods

The Value of Sprouts
Growing Your Own Sprouts
Uses for Sprouts
The Power of Associations with Family and Friends
Recipe – Hiziki Ginger Cabbage Salad
Recipe – Seed Cheese
Recipe – Nut Ricotta Cheese
Recipe – Garlic Dill Dip
Recipe – Tomato Basil Sauce

Day 8 Food Combinations that Give You Everything You Need for Total Health
Organic Fruits and Vegetables – Why Spend More? Because You're Worth It!
Organic Gardening in Your Yard or on Your Patio
Becoming Self-Sufficient
Goals, Faith and Belief
Deep Breathing – The Air of Life
Recipe – Fermented Nut and Seed Dishes
Recipe – Walnut Steak
Recipe – Apple Waldorf Salad
Recipe – Rejuvelac Champagne

Day 9 Specialty Foods
Visualization and Meditation
Do What You Love to Do
Discovering Your Purpose
Attracting What You Want
Discussing Changes You Already See
Staying Focused on What You Really Want
Persistence
Recipe – Pesto Sauce
Recipe – Smoky Dip with Veggies
Recipe – Veggie Lasagna
Packing Vege-Kraut

Day 10 Decorating Food to Make It Look Like a Work of Art
Decorating a Beautiful Party Table
Presentation of Living Foods Lifestyle Certificates of Course Completion

Summary of the Living Foods Lifestyle
The Physiology of Excellence
Staying Focused on Your Goals
The Party: A Celebration of Your Accomplishments with
    Family and Friends
What to Do Next!
Recipe – Nori Rolls
Recipe – Pesto Pasta

Recipes may be added or deleted according to the season and availability of organic ingredients. The recipes listed are just a few examples of those you will learn in class.

WHAT YOU'LL RECEIVE

As part of the 10-Day Training Program, every student will:

- Receive training in food preparation including hands-on instruction.
- Learn many recipes including the main healing foods, gourmet dishes and special quick-and-easy recipes.
- Become familiar with kitchen equipment.
- Enjoy the recipes you prepare and feast on a complete meal of Living and raw foods lovingly prepared by staff and student volunteers. (The four main foods for healing, Energy Soup, Rejuvelac, Vege-Kraut and Wheatgrass Juice, will be the center-piece complemented by delicious gourmet recipes.)
- Soak and sprout nuts, seeds, berries and grains and grow wheatgrass.
- Experience lessons designed to help you heal your body, mind and spirit.
- Learn the emotional reason behind each different symptom or disease and how to change your thoughts so you can heal.
- Receive a training manual with in-depth recipes, lessons and guides to healing the body, mind and spirit.
- Receive colon care equipment including an enema bag and plunge syringe, plus an in-class demonstration of how to use this equipment. (It's entertaining and fun!)
- Become a lifetime member of the Living Foods Institute so you

may participate in free support groups and the volunteer work-study program.

- Have access to the chi machine.
- Receive Brenda's book, **The Living Foods Lifestyle**, to support you in your healing journey.
- Be eligible for a lifetime student discount on equipment, books, supplies and food.
- Receive a Certificate of Completion for the Living Foods Lifestyle.

* We reserve the right to add or delete items.

Please call for the most up-to-date information regarding prices, dates, times and locations of classes. Also, for more information about products, please contact us at:

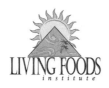

Living Foods Institute
1530 Dekalb Ave., NE, Suite E
Atlanta, GA 30307
Tel. (404) 524-4488
     (800) 844-9876
Fax: (404) 524-3932
www.livingfoodsinstitute.com

ACKNOWLEDGEMENTS

I thank God for the opportunity I have been given to help and teach others. I know God is working in me around me and through me for good. I am blessed by so many beautiful and loving people who have come into my life because of this work. I know that in this work God has a well-designed plan for healing the world one person at a time and that I am an instrument of God to do this work. It is an honor and a privilege.

I acknowledge each of my students for having the courage to step out of their comfort zones and change their thoughts and actions so they can change their worlds. It takes tremendous strength to change old habits. I honor and salute every one of you as you make your journey to spiritual awareness and total and perfect health. It is my privilege to teach you. You, in turn, have taught me much, for which I am eternally grateful. Thank you for enriching my life. I love each and every one of you.

I thank my beautiful, sweet mother, Myrtle Burnette, who has always been a tremendous light of love and beauty in my life. Thank you, Mama, for always helping me with whatever I needed. You have always supported me in all that I have done. I am truly blessed to have such an angel for a mother. The sacrifices you made for me throughout my life have not gone unnoticed or unappreciated. I thank God for you every single day, and I am so fortunate to have you in my life. I love you dearly.

I thank my fabulous husband who loves me unconditionally and who has always been there for me – to help me with anything I've needed. Ken, you have brought me incredible joy, and I am blessed to have you as my life's companion and partner. Thank you for the understanding and support you have willingly and lovingly given me. Thank you for building a beautiful Living Foods Center for all of us to enjoy, and, of course, thank you for always coming to the rescue to fix whatever needs fixing. You are my special "Mr. Fix-It." I love and adore you. Thank you for standing beside me and working with me every day to make the Living Foods Institute a continued success.

I thank my wonderful son, Richard Byrd, whose love and support in establishing the Living Foods Institute has been such a blessing. Thank you, Rich, for always being behind me and taking care of all the details – small and large – so I can spread the Living Foods message to the world. Your loving support means so much to me. As you move forward to pursue your own dream of a financial planning business, I wish you continued success and much joy and happiness. I am the luckiest mother alive to have such a beautiful, caring, supportive son. I love you so much!

I thank Shannon Wilder, my sweet, smart, capable editor. Thank you for your skills, your support and the love with which you edited this book. I could never thank you enough for your organization of our training manual and for your input into this project. You are a joy to be around with such a sweet and loving spirit. I love you and thank you from the bottom of my heart.

Thank you, Joanne Trinh, for preparing such delicious Living Foods in our Living Foods Kitchen. Joanne, you are truly a gift from God and we are blessed to have you as a part of our team. Your patience and understanding are admired by all. You add so much more than just ingredients into your recipes, you add your love as well. You are a true friend and constant support to me, and I love you for it.

Thank you, Alston Anderson, for the wonderful design work and beautiful cover. Thank you for your intelligent and professional input and your love and interest in this project. You have a beautiful light shining from within you and you are such a support for the Living Foods Institute and for me. I am blessed by your friendship.

Thank you, Jane Holmes, for the wonderful photography for the book, but most of all thank you for your never-ending friendship and love. For many years you have been my true friend and confidant. You have given me love and support in all areas of my life and have always been there when I have needed you. Your contributions and teachings in our emotional healing workshops are so appreciated by me and all of the students who participate. You are such a special blessing to me.

Thank you to Living Foods Institute student Steve Miller of Classic Landscapes (Fine Gardening Without Chemicals), for providing the beautiful organic flowers for the book cover photo shoot. You are so special, loving and giving. Your warm heart and caring personality are such a gift. I appreciate you and your wonderful mission to make our gardens and landscapes beautiful and without chemicals.

Thank you, Dr. Kathryn Lawson, my holistic chiropractor, for the incredible healing I have experienced. There are not adequate words to truly express the great and positive impact you have had on me and my healing journey. Thank you for helping me uncover the true, buried emotions behind each of my challenges and to help me to release and heal each one. You brought me quickly forward in my healing and have empowered me beyond imagination. All I can say is, Wow!

Thank you, my dear friend and healer, Faith Walker. You have given me wonderful therapy and beautiful, healing massages. Your touch has relaxed and rejuvenated me. You have a most wonderful gift as a healer and are one of the most loving and caring people I have ever known. I cannot thank you enough for all the times you have "saved" me and for how you have given so freely to all of our students. You are beautiful!

Thank you to all the volunteers who help us at the Living Foods Institute. You do such a fabulous job working with us and helping us with the many tasks required to run a successful Center. Also, thanks to the volunteers, Diana Stockton and Kathy Cromartie who helped to proofread my book.

Thank you to all of the health practitioners who come to the Living Foods Institute to teach and empower our students to go forward in their healing journeys.

INDEX

Cooked to death 69 A B